The Hormone Decision

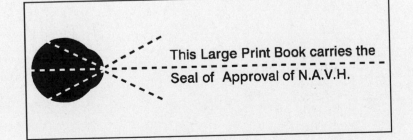

THE HORMONE DECISION

UNTANGLE THE CONTROVERSY; UNDERSTAND YOUR OPTIONS; MAKE YOUR OWN CHOICES

TARA PARKER-POPE

THORNDIKE PRESS

A part of Gale, Cengage Learning

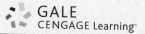

GALE
CENGAGE Learning™

Detroit • New York • San Francisco • New Haven, Conn • Waterville, Maine • London

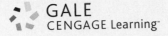

Thorndike Press® Large Print Health, Home and Learning.
The text of this Large Print edition is unabridged.
Other aspects of the book may vary from the original edition.
Set in 16 pt. Plantin.
Printed on permanent paper.

LIBRARY OF CONGRESS CATALOGING-IN-PUBLICATION DATA

Parker-Pope, Tara.
    The hormone decision : untangle the controversy, understand your options, make your own choices / by Tara Parker-Pope. — Large print ed.
        p. cm.
    Includes bibliographical references and index.
    "The text of this Large Print edition is unabridged".
    ISBN-13: 978-1-4104-0604-0 (hardcover : alk. paper)
    ISBN-10: 1-4104-0604-0 (hardcover : alk. paper)
    1. Menopause — Hormone therapy — Popular works. 2. Large type books. I. Title.
RG186.P39 2007
618.1'7506—dc22   2007051963

Published in 2008 by arrangement with Rodale Press, Inc.

Printed in the United States of America
1 2 3 4 5 6 7 12 11 10 09 08

For my mom. I miss you.

CONTENTS

INTRODUCTION

Confused about hormones? It's no wonder.
For years, women have taken prescription hormones to boost their health before, during, and after that important life transition called menopause. It's a time when hot flashes, mood swings, and other changes announce that our ovaries are shifting gears and getting out of the baby business. As our natural estrogen and progesterone levels wax and wane, hormones in a pill have been a way to calm the hormonal chaos going on inside our bodies and give us much-needed relief from the vexing symptoms of menopause.

But after years of feeling good about hormone drugs, today women are scared to death. Newspapers, magazines, and television shows are filled with frightening reports about menopause hormones and studies linking them to heart attack, stroke, breast cancer, and other health worries. The

latest research has seemed to contradict decades of scientific study in which hormone drugs appeared to protect women's hearts. The conflicting reports about hormones, heart attacks, and hot flashes are enough to leave your head spinning.

But you don't have to be confused anymore. The purpose of this book is to tell you the facts about menopause hormones and the science behind all the recent publicity. Once you look behind the headlines, you'll realize that much of what you've read about menopause hormones has been misleading or just plain wrong.

The reason the hormone debate seems so confusing is that the medical community itself is confused about hormones. Every new hormone study seems to contradict the previous one. But in recent years, scientists have begun to make sense of much of the new hormone research. They've discovered that while the answers aren't always simple, they aren't nearly as scary as we've been led to believe. Unfortunately, most of these new insights haven't been widely reported, and many women and doctors haven't gotten the message. No single study can provide all the answers we need about menopause hormones. But every new study, every new report — no matter how bad or good the

news seems at first — is simply one more small piece of the puzzle.

This book will help you see how all these pieces fit together. It will serve as a step-by-step guide to understanding the hormones made by your body and the hormones made by drug companies. It will also shed light on the controversial history of hormone science and hormone drugs, giving you insight into the historical context that frames today's debate.

In these pages, you will embark on a head-to-toe tour of how hormones affect various parts of your body, based on not one but hundreds of scientific studies. You will learn what scientists know about how hormones affect your heart, your brain, your bones, your breasts, and every other imaginable body part. You will learn about the laboratories at Wake Forest University where for years, scientists have studied how hormones influence the heart health of monkeys. You will visit 120,000 nurses who have selflessly given their time and their personal health information to create one of the largest and most important studies ever of women's health. From the "horse pee" farms of Canada to pharmacies that peddle so-called "natural hormones" — you will understand the risks and benefits of all the various

products now touted as options to relieve menopausal symptoms.

Most important, you will get an insider's view of the now-famous Women's Health Initiative (WHI), the government-sponsored study of more than 27,000 women that has produced the most-frightening reports about the risks and benefits of menopause hormones. As the health columnist for the *Wall Street Journal,* I have followed this groundbreaking study since the first WHI hormone results were announced in the summer of 2002. Since then, I have conducted extensive interviews with the scientists, medical doctors, and government health officials behind the WHI and spent countless hours poring over hundreds of pages of detailed scientific papers explaining the research. The WHI is the biggest-ever clinical trial evaluating women's health, and the data it has produced have proved exceedingly difficult to interpret. What has emerged is a far more complicated hormone story than has been reflected in the headlines and sound bites that appeared after the WHI results were first announced. In reading this book, you will see the miscalculations and the missteps that the government and the WHI scientists have made along the way and how these decisions and

hurdles have clouded the debate and confused women.

In July 2002, many of the scientists behind the WHI told women to stop taking hormones because of worries about heart attacks and breast cancer. Today, after a closer look at the study data, these same scientists have realized that hormones are likely safe — and in some cases, possibly even protective — for women seeking relief from menopausal symptoms. The WHI researchers continue to mine the data that are still pouring in from this important study. And some of the WHI's top scientists are pursuing new research, trying to determine if there is a window of opportunity when menopause hormones are safest and most effective for women.

Over the years, many of my readers have asked me whether hormones are good for you or bad for you. Unfortunately, there's no simple, one-size-fits-all answer to that question. A woman who chooses hormones must weigh all the risks and benefits. And a woman who chooses not to take hormones — opting instead for other drugs or treatments, or nothing at all — has her own set of risks and benefits to consider. Whatever the decision, the bottom line is that a woman needs to be fully informed about all

13

the various medical technoloies available to her throughout her life. And she needs to be smart about the hormone decision. A woman who decides not to take hormones needs to do it with the same level of information and insight as the woman who chooses to use these drugs.

Because hormones aren't right for every woman, this book also includes information about other treatment options for menopausal women. The right answer for you depends on a variety of factors, including your own personal health risks and fears, the severity of your symptoms, your family history, and your own values about medicine, and your personal health. The good news is that today, the women now approaching menopause will be the first generation to benefit from the recent science.

Our mothers and grandmothers experienced menopause with little information about the changes in their bodies or the options available to them. They had no solid research data about the risks and benefits of hormones on which to base their decisions — only hype, conjecture, and speculation. You will be among the first generation of women to make a truly informed decision about the best choices during this important

transition in life. In the end — whether you choose prescription hormones, herbal remedies, or nothing at all — the hormone decision you make will be the right one for you.

■ ■ ■ ■

PART ONE:
UNTANGLING THE
CONTROVERSY

■ ■ ■ ■

1
HORMONE CONFUSION: MAKING SENSE OF THE HEADLINES

On the morning of July 9, 2002, women woke up to some shocking news. The menopause hormones they had been taking to cope with hot flashes, improve their sex lives, strengthen their bones, and possibly help their hearts had turned against them. Or so it seemed.

The subject dominating the news over the next few days was the Women's Health Initiative (WHI), a government-funded study of 27,347 women that had set out to determine whether menopause hormones helped prevent heart disease, a benefit widely ascribed to hormone use. As it turned out, in the first group of 16,608 women to be tracked, the menopause hormone Prempro — a mixture of estrogens and a progestin made by pharmaceutical giant Wyeth — hadn't helped. Women in this study who used the drug had more heart attacks and breast cancer than non-

hormone users. They also had fewer hip fractures and lower risk of colon cancer, but that potential good news was eclipsed by the heart and breast worries. Government health officials had decided the risks to the women in the study outweighed the benefits, prompting them to take the unusual step of stopping the main part of the hormone study early.[1]

Within days of notifying the study participants, they held a hastily organized press conference to alert the public. Dozens of reporters attended the event at the National Press Club. Officials from the National Institutes of Health (NIH) and the study investigators hit the morning talk show circuit and evening news programs to spread the word.

The impact was immediate and lasting. For years, doctors had told us that menopause hormones protected women's hearts. Now some of the same doctors were on national television telling us just the opposite. Even veteran newscasters seemed flummoxed by the results, which ran counter to long-held beliefs about menopause hormones. "I tell you — women gotta go insane today," exclaimed CNN newswoman Paula Zahn.[2]

Hormone sales plummeted overnight as

women threw out their pills. Going off hormones cold turkey made them miserable, but they were too scared to keep taking them, certain that heart attacks, breast cancer, and all sorts of other maladies were now lurking around the corner, all because of hormones. They tried calling their doctors for guidance, but the phones were busy, swamped with other equally terrified patients trying to make sense of the news. The women who got through eventually discovered that their own doctors didn't really know what to do either.

HYPING THE RESULTS

Over the ensuing weeks and months, it became apparent that something had gone terribly wrong with the WHI. Screaming matches and name-calling erupted at medical meetings. WHI investigators stood firm in their findings. The researchers believed that the real problem was not the study itself but the fact that hormone proponents had spent years touting the benefits of the drugs and now just didn't want to admit they were wrong.

Meanwhile, longtime believers in menopause hormones were convinced that the study itself was somehow flawed and that this was all an effort to undermine hor-

mones in favor of other types of drug treatments. Some of the nation's top menopause experts accused the WHI scientists of misinterpreting the study data in a way that created hysteria and hype.

So who was right?

Years later, scientists are just starting to make sense of the data that have emerged from this important study. Many questions still aren't answered. But looking back, it's clear that the government's quick interpretation of the study and alarmist public announcements did mislead millions of American women. Subsequent analyses of the WHI hormone data have shown that the findings are not as clear-cut as they seemed on that summer day in Washington, DC.

A closer look at the study shows that key mistakes were made in the early design of the WHI. For a variety of reasons, the WHI was not a study of menopause but evolved as a study of older women who took menopause hormones. The average woman in the WHI was 63, and most women in the study started taking hormones at least 10 years past menopause. This fundamental flaw in the study design means the data are of limited use in trying to understand the full range of risks and benefits to the typical user of menopause hormones.

Today, the typical woman who is considering hormone therapy is in her late forties or early fifties. She's just beginning to experience the hormonal turmoil — the hot flashes, mood swings, and other changes — associated with the menopausal transition. Although few women in this age group were studied in the WHI, these are the women who have been most frightened and affected by the research.

In telling the public about the study findings, government health officials overstepped the scientific boundaries of the research, and the result was a much-exaggerated interpretation of the WHI data. One of the most egregious examples was the statement by Jacques Rossouw, MD, who at the time was acting director of the WHI. "The results have broad applicability," Dr. Rossouw told a roomful of reporters. "The study found no differences in risk by prior health status, age, or ethnicity."[3] Subsequent scientific analyses, published in respected medical journals, showed that the data are far more complex than that. They strongly suggest that the results probably don't apply to every woman.

As mentioned earlier, most of the women in the WHI started taking hormones at least 10 years past menopause; some were even

20 years past menopause. Think about this. Most of the women in the WHI were long past the hot flashes, sleep problems, mood changes, and other symptoms that persist throughout the menopausal transition. They were done with it. But for the sake of the WHI, they started taking hormones anyway. The study clearly showed it's not a good idea to begin taking hormones a decade or more after menopause, but what about those women who start sooner? A closer look at both WHI hormone studies — one of estrogen plus progestin, the other of estrogen alone — shows that the women in the studies who took hormones closest to the time of menopause had far fewer health risks and may have even received additional heart protection from hormone use.[4, 5]

What does all this mean to you today, as you are struggling with your own hormone decision? In trying to understand the latest science on hormones, it's important to know that most of the recent headlines and news reports came straight from the data in the WHI — and much of the current thinking about hormones has been shaped by the government's initial announcements about the first phase of the study. Virtually everything you will read about menopause hormones for the next decade will be based on

the WHI.

What has become increasingly clear is that the WHI is not the definitive word on menopause hormones. The WHI simply wasn't designed to give us information about most of the women who use hormones to treat the symptoms of menopause. Top government health officials and many WHI investigators have become sharply critical of that July 2002 press conference that has scared so many women about hormones. "It was presented in a very dramatic fashion," says Barbara Alving, former acting director of the National Heart, Lung, and Blood Institute (NHLBI), who temporarily took over the WHI after the first results were announced. "There should have been less drama and more thought. What we learned is that we need to work much better in the communication of risk, so people can understand it."

None of this means that the WHI is a bad study. Far from it. The WHI is the result of years of painstaking and high-quality scientific research. It is packed with voluminous amounts of valuable data. Dismissing this research would also be a disservice to women. The WHI has given us more information about hormones than we've ever had before.

The challenge is trying to figure out what the WHI really taught us and what it didn't. To make sense of it, you have to go back to the beginning, to the early days when the WHI was just an idea and scientists were trying to come up with the best way to learn about the risks and benefits of menopause hormones.

HORMONES AND THE HEART

At the time the WHI was devised, doctors had set out to answer the question of whether hormones could protect women from heart attacks. Answering this question was the primary purpose of the study. In 1991 when the WHI started, the thinking about women, hormones, and heart health was very different than it is today. The medical community was (and, actually, still is) heavily influenced by a major study from Harvard researchers called the Nurses' Health Study, which has followed the habits, health, and lifestyles of 120,000 nurses. In 1985,[6] health surveys from 32,000 of the nurses provided researchers with some surprising and convincing data. The nurses who used menopause hormones were 50 percent less likely to have a heart attack than nurses who didn't use hormones. A follow-up study in 1991[7] confirmed the

findings.

The data generated much excitement in the women's health community. An intervention that could lower heart attack risk by half would have a dramatic impact on women's health and save tens of thousands of lives. There was a lot of excitement, but there were also caveats. The Nurses' Health Study wasn't a clinical trial where one treatment is tested against a placebo. It was an observational study — that is, the women's habits and health were subjected to scientific scrutiny, but the women themselves were making their own choices about treatments, exercise, and medical checkups. Scientists know that you have to be cautious about how you interpret data from such a study. Were the nurses having fewer heart attacks because they used hormones? Or were the nurses who used hormones just healthier to start with? The type of woman who seeks out hormone treatment likely is getting regular medical care and is proactive about her health in other ways as well.

The question was: Do hormones keep you healthy? Or do healthy women use hormones?

Despite the scientific community's reservations about the Nurses' Health Study data, doctors and patients got excited about

hormones. Physicians began routinely prescribing them to women — and not just to those who were coping with menopause symptoms. The thinking was that if hormones helped protect women's hearts, they should be given to the women who needed them most — those who were older and at the highest risk for suffering a heart attack.

It seemed to make sense at the time, but today, it seems nothing short of bizarre. We're talking about 75-year-old women, long past menopause with no symptoms whatsoever, walking out of their doctors' offices with prescriptions for menopause hormones.

LOOKING FOR ANSWERS

In 1991, Bernadine Healy, MD, the first woman to run the NIH, decided to embark on a major clinical trial of women's health issues. The study would look at hormone use, calcium and vitamin D supplementation, and low-fat diets, attempting to measure how these interventions affected women's risk of heart attack, breast and colon cancer, and osteoporosis, among other things. But in designing the hormone portion of the study, the study investigators had two big problems.

First, most women who take hormones to

treat the symptoms of menopause are in their late forties or early fifties. They typically are healthy. For most of them, it will be at least 20 years before any signs of heart trouble show up. In science, it's expensive to study a healthy young woman. The reason: A study of healthy menopausal women would take years — possibly decades — before the women would be old enough to start having enough heart attacks to produce any meaningful results.

To find out if hormones would lower heart attack risk, the scientists needed to study women who would actually have heart attacks. If hormones helped, then women in the placebo group (the study participants who weren't taking the real drug) would have more heart attacks than women taking hormones. But nobody in the study would have heart attacks if they weren't old enough to be at risk for heart trouble to begin with. Although men see a jump in heart attack risk around age 45, a woman's heart attack risk doesn't start to rise until age 55. Most women won't face any heart risk until they are past 70.

But the WHI investigators couldn't wait 20 years for a 50-year-old menopausal woman to have a heart attack. They wanted and needed the data much sooner than that.

In order for the WHI to examine the heart effects of hormones, the investigators needed to recruit women who were at risk for heart attacks in the next 5 to 10 years. And they needed some of the women in the study to actually have heart attacks. If their theory held up, more heart attacks would happen to the women who weren't taking hormones.

The second dilemma was due to the fact that menopause can produce a variety of distressing symptoms — hot flashes, sleep disturbances, bleeding irregularities, and numerous other complaints. The WHI investigators worried that if they tried to look at the effect of hormones on women in the throes of menopause, the study probably wouldn't get far. That's because this was to be a random, blinded, controlled clinical trial — considered the gold standard of scientific research. It meant that some women would get real hormones, and some would get placebos. And nobody — not the women, not the doctors treating them, not the investigators — was supposed to know who was getting what.

But imagine if you were a menopausal woman in the study. You are waiting for an appointment with study doctors, and other women from the study also happen to be

there. These women are relaxing, flipping through magazines, or dozing in the waiting room. Meanwhile, you are flushed and miserable. Your body is dripping with sweat, you can't sleep, and your bleeding has become so irregular that you position yourself right next to the ladies' room. It will take you about 2 seconds to figure out that the other women are getting the real thing, and the pill you've been taking every day is a fake. And the moment you walk into the exam room, your doctor will figure it out too. So much for a random, blinded study.

Study investigators anticipated that women with bothersome menopause symptoms would quickly drop out of the study if the pills they took didn't relieve their symptoms. The only way to solve the problem was to study hormone use in women who didn't have menopause symptoms. Today, it may sound silly to give a menopause hormone to a woman who's not experiencing menopause symptoms. But at the time, the widespread belief was that hormones helped protect the heart. It didn't matter if you had symptoms or not; many doctors would put you on hormones anyway — just like they now advise men over age 50 to take a daily aspirin. Hormones were viewed as an all-purpose wonder drug. In

fact, so strong was the belief in hormones that some WHI investigators worried that it would be unethical to give some women a placebo.

A CRITICAL ERROR

So here is the dilemma faced by the WHI design team: How do you study the connection between heart attacks and hormones in a way that women won't figure out whether they are getting the real hormone or a placebo? And how do you study the drugs in the shortest possible time, making sure that enough heart attacks happen in order to produce meaningful data?

The answer was to study older women. Older women have heart attacks. Older women don't have menopause symptoms. Problem solved.

But really, looking back, it's clear that this is where the WHI's problems started.

This major national study of menopause hormones was conducted primarily in older women who weren't experiencing menopause. As mentioned earlier, the average age of the WHI participants was 63. That's 10 to 15 years older than the typical woman who seeks advice about menopause hormones.

Further increasing the need to enroll older

women was the fact that the WHI was supposed to study more than hormones. Other parts of the WHI were looking at hip fracture risk among women who take calcium and the effect of a low-fat diet on breast cancer risk. Many of the women in the calcium and diet studies would also be used in the hormone study. As with heart attacks, hip fractures and breast cancer are more likely to occur in older women.

Initially, investigators decided to recruit an equal number of women in their fifties, sixties, and seventies. But as the scientists began the complex statistical calculations necessary to design a study, they realized that the risk of breast cancer among women ages 50 to 54 was actually higher than the risk of a heart attack. Because this was to be primarily a study of heart attacks, the decision was made to further reduce the number of 50- to 54-year-old participants. As a result, of the 27,347 women in both of the WHI hormone studies, only 3,425 were under age 55.

At the time, some investigators raised questions about whether this was the best way to design a study. Ultimately, though, the WHI team — along with the rest of the medical community — was convinced that the study would show hormones to be good for women at any time during or after menopause. They didn't realize that adding so many older women to the study group had potentially doomed the research before it even started.

The WHI Begins

So by the time the WHI got underway, the government had designed a study of menopause hormones that wasn't about menopause at all. Younger women experiencing menopause symptoms were largely excluded from the research. Only about 14 percent of those in the study actually had moderate to severe hot flashes. In fact, WHI wasn't even designed to measure relief from hot flashes, which is the primary benefit of menopause hormones.

At the time, none of this seemed like a fatal flaw. All these decisions were made not to undermine the WHI but to strengthen it. The thinking was that choosing mostly older women with no symptoms would improve the study, giving it more statistical power and the ability to generate useful information more quickly.

Once the study started, another big problem developed. A lot of the women weren't consistently taking their study pills. One theory is that the women were simply overburdened by the demands of the research. Taking part in any clinical trial is time-consuming, but many of the women in the hormone segment of the WHI were also taking part in the calcium or diet study. The problem is, the WHI was based on several key statistical assumptions. If too many women dropped out or stopped taking the treatment, it would change the statistical validity of the data that emerged. By the end of the study, nearly half of the women in both hormone trials had stopped taking their pills.[8, 9]

In 1997, the first signs that the WHI wasn't going as planned began to surface. Although all the doctors and patients in the study were "blinded" — meaning they didn't know who was receiving the real hormone pills — a select group of WHI officials did have access to some data. A safety-monitoring board was tracking the overall differences between the hormone users and the placebo group every 6 months. The first hint of trouble showed up in the fall of 1997, when the safety group noticed more health problems among hormone users.[10] Given the nature of scientific research, this could have been just a hiccup. Differences between treatment groups can move up and down all the time; sometimes, it takes years for a distinct pattern to emerge. But this pattern didn't change.

In 2000, the WHI sent letters to women taking part in the study, alerting them that hormone users seemed to have a higher risk of heart attacks, blood clots, and strokes, but that the trend appeared to be attenuating over time. Another letter was sent in 2001, telling the women that the balance of risks and benefits remained uncertain.[11]

What this means is that the NIH knew for at least 2 years that the older hormone users in the WHI were experiencing more health problems than those in the placebo group were. At the same time, other studies had already begun to show that the hormone story was different than once thought. In 1998, for example, a study called HERS (which stands for the Heart and Estrogen/ Progestin Replacement Study) had found that older women with existing heart disease weren't helped by hormone use.[12]

Although the WHI was supposed to continue until 2005, the safety board decided to stop the estrogen and progestin arm of the study in May 2002. Even so, the government sat on the information for another few months as it worked to write up the data and have the results published in the *Journal of the American Medical Association*. NIH officials didn't want the news leaking out and kept most of the details a secret, even from many of the WHI investigators themselves.

When it was time to release the news, however, the NIH wanted to make a splash. The NHLBI, which oversaw the WHI, worked hard to get media attention for the WHI study. Dr. Rossouw, the physician in charge of the WHI when the results were first announced, has since told me that the NHLBI was intentionally going for "high impact" when it called the press conference in Washington, DC. Dr. Rossouw and other NIH officials knew that important health announcements could get lost in the shuffle of daily news events, but they didn't want this study ignored. The goal, says Dr. Rossouw, was to shake up the medical establishment and change the thinking about hormones.

Looking back, it was overkill. For some time prior to the WHI's release, other studies had already been showing that hormones didn't help women who already had heart disease. The findings of these studies were barely noticed by the media, but medical practice had started to change. To be sure, there remained a general belief that a woman's heart health does benefit from hormone use, but the practice of prescribing hormones to older women to protect their hearts was already on the decline. In 1998, an estimated 72 percent of doctors who prescribed hormones said that one reason for doing so was to protect women's hearts. By 2002, before the WHI results were released, the number had dropped to about 16 percent.[13] Clearly, most doctors had already gotten the message that there were likely better ways to protect a woman's heart than with hormones.

The problem is that in its effort to further change thinking about hormones and heart risk, the NHLBI ended up scaring every woman who ever used hormones. In fact, the biggest misstep of the WHI is the alarmist way in which government health officials announced the first hormone study results.

Harvard researchers recently analyzed the differences in publicity surrounding the WHI compared with other studies on menopause hormones. In particular, they looked at news coverage before and after the 1998 HERS report, the study that showed hormone use might be risky for older women with heart disease. They compared the way the press covered HERS in the months before and after the study with the news coverage before and after the announcement of the WHI results. Both studies showed hormones to be risky for older women. But the number of articles about the WHI and menopause hormones published during the month of July 2002 was eight times greater than the number of articles published before and after the HERS trial.[14]

The NIH got the media blast it had hoped for. The main problem with this approach is that even the most-experienced scientists need time to mull the details of such a massive clinical trial. Most of the time, such studies are published in medical journals, and doctors debate the findings among themselves. Eventually they reach a consensus that gets translated to patients. But none of this happened with the WHI. The study results were trumpeted to the media, doctors, and patients all at the same time. It's taken veteran researchers years to start to make sense of these data — and there are still many more questions being asked. But women didn't have the luxury to mull the results. They were scared and forced to make fast decisions about their health.

In the years since the first WHI results were announced, I found myself increasingly questioning the way the NIH and others had interpreted the data from this important study of women's health. What was so troubling was that the NHLBI was not at all consistent in how it viewed the results. Trends that showed hormones might be bad for women were highlighted, even if the data weren't statistically sound. Trends that showed hormones might be beneficial were often ignored or downplayed.

For instance, the WHI heart data from the estrogen and progestin trial missed statistical significance by the slimmest of margins. Still, women were warned of a 24 percent higher heart attack risk. On the other hand, when the estrogen-only study showed the good news that estrogen might *lower* breast cancer risk by 20 percent, the NHLBI didn't tout the finding. Instead, the headline on the government press release said only that there was "no increased risk of breast cancer with estrogen alone."[15] The NHLBI seemed to have a different standard for bad hormone news than it did for good hormone news.

Even though the NHLBI has been inconsistent in how it interprets the WHI data, that doesn't mean we shouldn't pay attention to the WHI. The raw data from the WHI represent a potential gold mine of information about women's health. We just have to be careful about what we conclude from it.

So What Did We Learn from the WHI?

The WHI revealed a lot about the risks and benefits of starting hormones at an older age. A woman who is past menopause shouldn't turn to hormones in hopes of boosting her health. The evidence is clear that starting hormones in older women long past menopause does more harm than good, increasing the risk of heart attacks, blood clots, strokes, and other health worries. Why this happens will be discussed throughout this book. But the bottom line is this: If you are long past menopause and have no symptoms, don't start taking hormones. This is the one area of hormone research where there really is no debate.

But what about younger women? It wasn't long after the WHI was stopped that people began to wonder if the results would have been different had more young women in the midst of the menopausal transition been included in the study. There's now a growing belief that the health effects of hormones vary depending on how old a woman is and where she is in her reproductive lifespan. The question is whether there is a window of opportunity in which hormone treatments can be safely used to treat menopause symptoms and possibly offer additional health benefits with minimal risks.

There are also questions raised by the WHI about the differences between women who use combination hormones (estrogen and progestin) and women who take only estrogen. Estrogen by itself increases the risk of uterine cancer. Adding progestin protects the uterus from estrogen's harmful effects. As a result, a woman with a uterus is advised to take a combination of estrogen and progestin. But a woman who has had a hysterectomy can take only estrogen to treat menopause symptoms. Because she no longer has a uterus and therefore isn't at risk for uterine cancer, she doesn't need progestin.

What has been so surprising about the WHI is the marked differences in the results between the study group taking combined hormones and the women taking only estrogen. It's the first time in history that anyone has attempted to measure the impact on a woman's body of adding progestin to the hormone mix. In fact, for women who have had a hysterectomy, the hormone decision in many ways will be made easier by the results of the WHI study. Women in the estrogen-only group actually had lower rates of heart attacks, breast cancer, and other ailments than women on the placebo. There was a slightly higher risk of stroke and blood clots — a finding that wasn't entirely surprising, given what was already known about the impact of hormones on clotting risks.

But the same caveats apply to the estrogen-only group. They were older women, long past menopause. Many researchers think it's likely that the results — particularly the risks — can't be easily translated to younger women. A close analysis of the data shows that many of the risks associated with estrogen use disappear among younger women close to menopause.

Indeed, in the years since the study results came out, it's become clear that little from the WHI can be extrapolated to the typical user of menopause hormones. But it can give us some important clues. Several researchers have begun to parse the data in an effort to better understand how hormones affect younger women. What has begun to emerge is evidence that menopause hormones are likely safe for women in the midst of the menopausal transition. Like every drug, menopause hormones carry risks, but they also may come with extra benefits. We will explore exactly what those are in future chapters, as we take a head-to-toe look at how hormones and menopause affect the heart, the breasts, the brain, and other body parts.

The WHI has helped illuminate the role of hormones in breast cancer, bone health, and other health concerns. It also has helped make sense of earlier hormone research, such as the Nurses' Health Study and other reports that have shown both risks and benefits from hormone use.

For better or worse, the WHI is now the main reference point for women and doctors when they discuss menopause as well as for scientists who work with hormones. It's only one study, but it's the biggest and one of the best, despite some of its inherent limitations and flaws. The WHI not only has shaped the way doctors and menopausal women think about hormones today, it also has altered the course of women's health for generations. That's why it's so important to learn more about the WHI — how it was conducted, how the data fit in with all the other research that came before it, and how it is helping scientists devise even better studies in the future.

The WHI has taught us that many of our assumptions about hormones have been wrong. It has raised new questions about the timing and duration of hormone use and the types of hormones — particularly the type of progestin — women should consider using. Perhaps most important, the WHI has taught us to ask better questions.

How do hormones affect women who take them to relieve menopausal symptoms? What about women who have had their ovaries removed and who take hormones to prevent premature menopause? What about older women who started hormones at menopause and are still taking them years later? If a woman stopped taking hormones because of health fears, is it safe for her to resume taking them to relieve ongoing symptoms? And what about alternatives to hormones — herbal supplements, antidepressants, and osteoporosis drugs? Are they a better choice for some women coping with the symptoms of menopause?

We don't know all the answers yet. But the good news is that we have more information than ever before about the risks and benefits of hormones, as well as other treatments used by women during menopause. For the first time in history, a woman can make an informed choice about whether to use menopause hormones to help her cope with the symptoms and challenges of this important time in her life.

But to make sense of any of this, you need to realize that much of what you've read about hormones in the past few years is

45

likely inaccurate. It's only recently that scientists have begun sorting through the WHI data and reconciling it with all the research that came before it. But the new findings about this important hormone study haven't generated the same headlines as the initial results.

While the scientific questions about the timing of hormone use and the potential for heart benefits continue to be debated, there is little debate now about the safety of hormones for women with menopause symptoms. Top menopause experts, heart experts, the NIH, and even the Food and Drug Administration all agree on this point. Since the initial WHI announcement, Dr. Rossouw and other NIH officials have softened their statements about hormones, noting that the drugs are a reasonable choice and likely safe for women to use for the short-term treatment of menopausal symptoms. They say it was never the intention of anyone at the NIH to frighten women about using hormones for this purpose.

That doesn't necessarily mean you should make the decision to use them. It means only that you need to go into this decision with an open mind, shaking loose your fears about heart attacks and other health problems that have scared so many women away from this treatment in recent years. The hormone decision is for you to make. You need to consider the facts, not the headlines.

So let's get started. The best place is at the beginning — looking back to a time when scientists first discovered hormones, the mysterious role they might play in women's health, and the first signs of the looming controversy that menopause and hormones would generate.

2
HORMONE HISTORY: THE PENDULUM SWINGS

To really make sense of recent hormone scares and headlines, it's important to know that we've been through it all before. The debate about whether hormones are good for you or bad for you has raged since 1898, when doctors first started grinding up cow ovaries and feeding them to women to help abate some of the more unpleasant aspects of menopause (not the least of which was the fact that they were advised to eat cow ovaries).

No other drugs in the history of medicine have been as consistently controversial as menopause hormones. For 100 years, various factions have argued that women were being either undertreated for menopause or overtreated for menopause. Over the course of several decades, women have been told to be wary of hormone treatments and then to embrace them, only to be told again about new health fears. At times, the feminist movement has argued both for and against hormone use. Some feminists believed hormones empowered women and freed them from debilitating menopause symptoms. At the same time, feminist critics derided the "medicalization" of menopause and the effort by the medical establishment to treat this natural phase in a woman's life as an illness.

For decades, the pendulum has swung back and forth in support and opposition to these drugs. It's still swinging today. In July 2002, officials from the National Institutes of Health (NIH) warned women about hormone dangers, claiming there was no reliably safe period to use them. Today, those same health officials tell women that they should be reassured by recent hormone studies and that the drugs are safe to use for relief of menopause symptoms.

Having a hard time keeping up? So is everyone else. Hormones have been subject to more mood swings than a menopausal woman.

What matters most to women and doctors is what we know *now* about hormones. And we know a lot more than we ever did. But to understand the headlines, the politics, and the latest science behind hormones, it's helpful to learn a little about the historical context of this polarizing debate.

MENOPAUSE: IS IT NATURAL OR A MODERN MISTAKE?

When a woman is young and fertile, the natural hormones made by her body rise and fall in a fairly predictable monthly cycle. A complex messaging system between the ovaries and the brain triggers ovulation, in which an egg is released, and the body readies itself to incubate a baby. If the egg isn't fertilized, the body adjusts, hormone levels drop, and the process starts over.

But as a woman ages and reproduction moves off the biological agenda, the ovaries shift gears. The ovulatory cycle, which generally occurs like clockwork in younger women, becomes less reliable. Eggs aren't consistently released from the ovaries, and the brain-ovary messaging system starts to break down. Initially, this can produce wild swings in a woman's estrogen levels, causing the most obvious signs of approaching menopause — hot flashes, irregular periods, mood swings, and other symptoms. Gradually, a woman stops ovulating altogether. Although the ovaries are done with egg production, they're still working. Eventually, the ovaries settle into a sort of maintenance mode, producing testosterone as well as low levels of estrogen and other hormones.[1,2]

A common argument against hormone use is that menopause is a natural process in a woman's life and shouldn't be treated as a disease that requires drug therapy. It is true that menopause is a natural process. But so is getting pregnant, and that never stopped women from wanting to control their fertility. We have accepted that women want to avail themselves of medical technology to control every aspect of their reproductive cycle. Women use birth control pills to prevent unwanted pregnancies. They use folic acid, sonograms, and fetal monitors to ensure a healthy baby. Women who can't get pregnant turn to fertility treatments. Once they are pregnant, many women opt for epidurals to help ease the pain of labor.

So why do the rules about medical technology suddenly change once a woman hits menopause? Women should be allowed to maintain as much control over their bodies at the end of their reproductive years as they had during the beginning and middle of the reproductive timeline. That doesn't mean every woman should choose hormones, but a woman who does decide to use hormones shouldn't be made to feel that the choice is an affront to nature.

At the same time, a common argument in favor of hormones is equally suspect. Hormone proponents often cite historical life-expectancy statistics to argue that menopause, in fact, is not natural. They suggest that women weren't supposed to live so long as to reach menopause, but that modern medicines like antibiotics and improvements in maternal health have increased life expectancy well beyond what nature intended. Since other medicines have helped us live longer than we were meant to, the argument goes, it's reasonable to turn to hormone drugs to stay healthy during a lifespan that has been artificially prolonged by science anyway.

But before you buy into this argument, think about the real meaning of life-expectancy data. Sure, many women throughout history have died in their thirties, forties, and fifties — either during childbirth or due to illness. But life expectancy is based on an average. Some people die very young, some die very old, and most die somewhere in between. There is lots of evidence that menopause isn't a modern accident and that women for thousands of years have outlived their reproductive life cycle. As Wulf Utian, MD, PhD, professor emeritus at Case University in Cleveland

and executive director of the North American Menopause Society, has noted, even the Bible recognizes that women can live past their fertile years.

There is a plausible evolutionary reason for menopause. It's called the "grandmother hypothesis." The basic idea is that a woman who keeps having children either can't take care of them all or simply would wear out under the stress of multiple childbirths. Evolution solved this problem by stopping a woman's reproductive cycle so that she could stop having her own children and tend to her grandchildren. That means that postmenopausal women aren't the by-product of modern medical advances; they are an evolutionary necessity.

WHAT EXACTLY IS MENOPAUSE?

Menopause, by definition, is a pause in your menses — the moment when your period stops, never to return. Women aren't aware of exactly when menopause occurs. We realize it has happened long after the fact. If it's been 12 months since your last period, then you are officially past menopause.

However, many women begin to notice changes before their periods stop for good. Changes in the timing of their menstrual cycles, irregular bleeding, and heavy periods are all signs that menopause is approaching. So too are hot flashes, changes in vaginal lubrication, fatigue, mood swings, and numerous other symptoms. But the magical 12-month dry spell signaling that menopause is officially over doesn't mean that the symptoms are over. Hormone levels in a woman's body can continue to fluctuate for a matter of months, and sometimes years, after her periods stop.

Various terms have been coined to describe the time in a woman's life before, during, and after menopause. Some doctors talk about "perimenopause" as the symptom-filled months or years before actual menopause. A woman who has stopped having periods is often referred to as "postmenopausal" — though this could describe a woman from age 50 to 100.

Most people typically fail to make any real distinction between perimenopause, menopause, and postmenopause. Instead, the word *menopause* is commonly used to describe the broad time frame during which women are experiencing the wide range of symptoms associated with fluctuating and declining estrogen levels. That's how I will use the term *menopause* in this book.

Menopause usually occurs naturally in women between ages 45 and 55. However, loss of estrogen can also occur if a woman has her ovaries removed surgically, if she undergoes cancer treatment, or if she experiences early menopause.

But Is It a Medical Problem?

It wasn't until the end of the 19th century that the medical community started paying close attention to menopause and all the physical and emotional changes that go with it. This was due in part to the emergence of gynecology and endocrinology as medical specialties. Surprisingly, it was a French physiologist's experiments on himself in 1889 that jump-started the scientific community's interest in menopause. The doctor reported feeling youthful and energetic after injecting himself with extracts from guinea pig and dog testes. Although the tests involved male reproductive organs, the experiments piqued scientific interest in a woman's "internal secretions" as well.[3]

In 1898, German doctors fed fresh cow ovaries to a young woman who was suffering from severe hot flashes after having her own ovaries removed. This led to a crude treatment called "organotherapy," which used pulverized ovaries from farm animals such as cows, sheep, and horses to relieve severe menopause symptoms.[4] The pharma-

ceutical company Merck developed Ova-
riin, a course brownish powder derived from
cow ovaries, for the treatment of menopause.[5] Although scientists had a strong
suspicion that the ovaries were somehow
intrinsically linked to menopause symptoms,
they didn't yet understand the roles estrogen
and progesterone play in a woman's reproductive health and the aging experience.

Despite a burgeoning interest in extracts
from reproductive organs, the notion of
"treating" menopause symptoms wasn't yet
widely embraced. Most doctors during the
early part of the 20th century didn't think
menopause was that big a deal. In 1903, a
paper in the *American Journal of Obstetrics*
claimed that the changes associated with
menopause "come about as gently as the
falling of the autumn leaves."[6]

According to University of Wisconsin
medical historian Judith A. Houck, PhD,
many physicians at the time believed that
women should talk to their doctors about
menopause, but they didn't view menopause
as a condition that required medical intervention. The belief was that women simply
needed information. Once they learned
about the changes in their bodies and the
various symptoms they would be experiencing as they aged, they would be less fearful

about the process and would start to feel better. While information is a powerful tool for achieving better health, the medical profession's practice at the time was essentially to dismiss women as nervous and anxious, rather than acknowledge the fact that many of them were suffering real physical symptoms associated with menopause.

It wasn't until 1929 that researchers in St. Louis and Germany first isolated a form of estrogen. Identifying the hormone was a scientific breakthrough, but researchers still hadn't found a practical way to use it as a treatment for women's health. The forms of estrogen that had been discovered weren't water soluble, which meant they couldn't be given as pills, so they were mixed with oil and given as injections, making them impractical for most women.[7]

That changed with the development of Emmenin, an oral estrogen that was marketed in the United States beginning in 1933. The problem with Emmenin was the source — urine from pregnant Canadian women. The product was popular, but making enough of it to keep up with demand was impossible. At about the same time as the development of Emmenin, German researchers discovered that the urine of pregnant horses also contained water-soluble estrogens that could ultimately be given in pill form. Ayerst, the drug company that made Emmenin, began looking at the medical and commercial potential of manufacturing a hormone treatment from a pregnant mare's urine. In 1939, the company processed its first gallon of horse urine. The result was a mixture of estrogen compounds that the company dubbed Premarin.[8]

The isolation of estrogen and a crude understanding of its chemical makeup also had led researchers to develop the first synthetic hormone, called diethylstilbestrol, or DES, in 1938. It was approved by the FDA in 1941 and marketed as a treatment for menopause.[9] It was an important milestone in hormone history because it marked the first time a hormone treatment was both practical (given in pill form) and affordable. (Later, DES was marketed as a way to prevent miscarriage, but eventually the agent was linked with a rare form of vaginal cancer.) A year after DES won FDA approval, the agency gave Ayerst permission to market Premarin for the treatment of menopause symptoms.

Despite the development of these potent new drugs, the medical community remained largely skeptical that there was any significant need to use hormones or anything else to help women cope with menopause. So by the 1950s, Ayerst had launched a massive education program among doctors, focusing on menopause, menopausal symptoms, and problems associated with declining estrogen levels in aging women.[10] This push to "educate" doctors about menopause hormones as a means of selling more hormone drugs raises a lot of questions about the role pharmaceutical companies played in shaping today's medical thinking about menopause. Critics claim that doctors and drug companies have colluded over the years to transform menopause from a natural biological condition into a disease requiring a pharmacological treatment. Clearly, the drug industry did help push the notion that menopause was a treatable condition and that hormones were the answer.

It's only fair to note that women, in general, were sadly neglected by the medical establishment in the first half of the 20th century (and many would argue they are still neglected today). Drug companies were trying to create a market for menopause hormones and convince doctors to prescribe them — but at the same time, doctors weren't listening to women's health concerns and complaints about the toll menopause symptoms could take. Many doctors didn't believe that menopause was a real health issue for women or that it was even a particularly meaningful experience. Sensing the growing importance of women's health and the impact of the women's rights movement, the drug industry started listening to women long before anyone else did. Whether they pushed the medical discussion and science in the right direction remains a matter of debate, but they clearly helped put the issue of women's health, menopause, and reproductive rights on the national agenda.

Notably, at the same time the first hormone drugs were coming to market, concerns about the link between hormones and certain cancers had begun to emerge, but they were largely ignored. According to Dr. Houck, by 1940, more than a dozen scientists had noted that synthetic and natural estrogens could cause cancer in female animals.[11] In 1947, Columbia University gynecologist Saul Gusberg, MD, who dedicated his career to the study of gynecological cancers, already had linked estrogen use to cancer of the endometrium, which is the lining of the uterus. Dr. Gusberg complained that estrogen was too freely prescribed and that its use was "promiscuous."[12] He was right about the risk of uterine cancer, but it would be nearly 30 years before women received adequate warnings about the problem.

Most doctors of the time felt that estrogen could offer short-term relief of menopause symptoms, but few advocated its long-term use. However, some doctors had just begun to tout the potential of estrogen to halt osteoporosis and heart disease, and the drum beats for long-term use of hormones began.

What's so fascinating about this early history of hormone therapy is that it so closely resembles some of the most recent controversy surrounding menopause hormones. Today, doctors still debate the cancer risk and potential impact of hormones on heart health, while noting that the treatments clearly boost bone health. Most health officials now recommend short-term use of hormones, although some proponents remain convinced that long-term use is safe and potentially beneficial for many women — proving once again that the more things change, the more they stay the same.

"FEMININE FOREVER"

The real turning point in the history of estrogen as a drug therapy came in 1963, when Robert Wilson, MD, a Brooklyn gynecologist, published an article in the *Journal of the American Geriatrics Society* in which he asserted that menopause was "Nature's defeminization." The article blamed the depletion of estrogen from a woman's body for causing various health problems, including osteoporosis. But the part of the article that had the most profound impact was his harsh description of women in the throes of menopause as emotionally disturbed, infirm, exhausted, and bereft of their femininity. Menopause, said Dr. Wilson, was a "supreme tragedy" and an "estrogen deficiency disease."[13] It was about time for somebody to acknowledge that menopause isn't always an easy experience for some women. But his description of women in menopause as shriveled up and decaying creatures is far off the mark.

The article made headlines, and journalists repeated Dr. Wilson's notions of menopause. In 1966, Dr. Wilson published the long version of his views in the book *Feminine Forever*. While *Feminine Forever* dramatically altered awareness of menopause (as well as the potential for the drug industry to capitalize on it), the timing of the book also helped to forever politicize the debate about hormones.

Feminine Forever was released at the budding of the women's rights movement. Many feminists at the time cited the lack of care for menopausal women as one of countless examples of the medical establishment neglecting the needs of women. In that sense, Dr. Wilson's book triggered a welcome focus on women's health, winning over some feminists. In addition, because menopausal women typically felt better using hormones, the treatment allowed them to remain in the workforce, care for their families, and contribute to society in other meaningful ways. Just as birth control pills could help women control their reproductive destiny, menopause hormones had the potential to allow women to continue to remain in control of their lives and bodies as they aged — truly a feminist ideal.

However, Dr. Wilson created a so-called "disease model" of menopause — describing it more as an illness than as a natural phase representing the end of a woman's reproductive cycle. He painted a picture of women as victims of their own biology who became useless to society if menopause was allowed to run its natural course.

As a result, the feminist movement was torn. In one respect, menopause hormones gave them control over their health and their bodies and served as an indicator that the medical establishment was finally paying much-needed attention to women's health. The question was whether this attention was welcome and useful or was simply a male-centered approach that undermined the complexity of a woman's natural aging process.

Dr. Wilson believed that hormone drugs were a "biological revolution" that meant women would never have to experience menopause. Menopause, wrote Dr. Wilson, was "completely preventable" and "curable" for women who used hormones.

Instead of being condemned to witness the death of their own womanhood during what should be their best years, they will remain fully feminine — physically and emotionally — for as long as they live. . . . The outward signs of this age-defying youthfulness are a straight-backed posture, supple breast contours, taut, smooth skin on face and neck, firm muscle tone, and that particular vigor and grace typical of a healthy female. At fifty, such women still look attractive in tennis shorts or sleeveless dresses.[14]

He went on to compare menopause with diabetes, noting that both are versions of a "deficiency disease" in which a missing substance — estrogen or insulin — can be replaced. He dedicated an entire chapter in his book to the notion that menopause is a form of female castration.

It makes no difference whether castration is brought about by removing the ovaries with a knife — as in their surgical removal — or whether the ovaries shrivel up and die as the result of menopause. In either case, the effect is the same; the woman becomes the equivalent of a eunuch.[15]

Feminine Forever is difficult reading in that it paints women as being wholly defined by their "femininity" and victims of their biology. At the same time, Dr. Wilson in many ways was an advocate for women and women's health in that he was issuing a clarion call for the medical establishment to pay attention to this medically important experience called menopause. He recognized the toll that hot flashes, vaginal atrophy, and other menopause symptoms could take on a woman (although he seemed to ignore the fact that only a minority of women suffer the most severe forms of these symptoms). He was correct in saying that loss of estrogen during menopause can lead to osteoporosis and the telltale "dowager's hump" that the disease could produce, and he acknowledged the mental toll and depression that can result from estrogen depletion. (But he wrongly dismissed outright concerns about the link between estrogen use and uterine cancer.)[16] Although Dr. Wilson's work has been criticized as sexist and patronizing, he viewed hormone therapy as the ultimate equalizer for women in a male-dominated society.

The technique of menopause prevention reaches far beyond the scope of any single life. It means that, for the first time in history, women may share the promise of tomorrow as biological equals of men. Specifically, they can remain able and active in mind and body for their entire lives.[17]

Dr. Wilson's book was a huge seller; following its publication, hormone use surged. Looking back, it's unfortunate that Dr. Wilson focused so much on femininity and the idea that a drug treatment could help make women more desirable to their husbands.

He had cast national attention on the need for menopause care, but his approach forever colored the discussion and the science about hormones. Rather than provoke a thoughtful examination of how doctors and medical technology might improve the quality of life for women as they aged, Dr. Wilson's views helped frame the feminist debate about menopause. Today, doctors and women's groups who are opposed to hormone use routinely cite some of Dr. Wilson's more outlandish and sexist statements, claiming that hormones are a direct result of an inherently misogynistic medical system.

Even so, hormones presented a dilemma for the feminist movement. At the same time that Dr. Wilson was promoting the benefits of hormones in the late 1960s, a new women's health movement was beginning to emerge. Feminists were divided on how to respond to this new drug treatment for women. The fact that women's needs during menopause had been ignored by the medical community for so long prompted some feminist writers to celebrate the development of hormones. Some feminists began to view estrogen therapy as a powerful weapon in the fight for women's liberation.[18]

In her book *Don't Change: A Biological Revolution for Women,* British journalist Wendy Cooper argued that menopause hormones gave women control over their bodies — the same control women had been fighting for over their reproductive health. Although critics had begun to assert that menopause was a natural phase in a woman's life and shouldn't be subject to medical intervention, Cooper noted that the same argument had been used to prevent women's access to contraception.[19] Other feminists argued that just because menopause is a "natural" phase in a woman's life, it shouldn't be confused with something that is desirable, any more than multiple childbirths, while natural, were typically not desirable to most women.[20]

Feminine Forever essentially framed the scientific and public discussion about menopause and hormones at a time when the feminist movement was just beginning to assert its considerable influence and political power. The confluence of these two events still influences the politics surrounding a woman's hormone decision today.

Another reason that hormones remain so politically charged is the shameful lack of research into their safety, risks, and benefits even as they were being widely and freely prescribed to women. Barbara Seaman, a longtime women's health advocate who for years has been raising important questions about hormone therapy, calls the unchecked use of menopause hormones "the greatest experiment ever performed on women."[21]

By current standards, hormone therapy was largely experimental throughout much of its history. Doctors, drug firms, and women themselves had pushed forward with hormone use despite any reliable evidence about safety or efficacy. Worse, the medical community dismissed early warnings about cancer concerns associated with the drugs.

In 1969, Seaman's book, *The Doctors' Case against the Pill,* helped change the debate about menopause hormones and women's health issues. The book delved into many of the unreported side effects of birth control pills and eventually led to congressional hearings and package inserts warning women about the risks associated with oral contraceptives. The book and the resulting controversy helped ignite a modern women's health movement that called for more and better research into safe practices, as well as adequate information about the risks associated with various drugs and medical procedures. In 1975, Seaman and several other women formed the National Women's Health Network, which among other initiatives launched a regular publication called *Taking Hormones and Women's Health.*

Also in 1975, two troubling studies appeared in the *New England Journal of Medicine.* Just like Dr. Gusberg had done nearly 30 years earlier, these studies showed a link between estrogen therapy and uterine cancer.[22] But this time, people paid attention. The *New England Journal* research, and the resulting cancer fear that spread among women, triggered a steep drop in hormone use. In 1975, doctors had written 28 million prescriptions for menopause hormones; the number dropped to just 15 million in 1980.

Doctors continued prescribing the drugs but not as freely, recommending them primarily for women with particularly distressing menopause symptoms. After 1975, women who opted for hormone drugs were advised to take lower doses for the shortest duration of time possible. (Notably, the advice was identical to that given in 2002 after the results of the recent Women's Health Initiative study were announced.)

The 1975 cancer scare had boosted interest in additional hormone research. In 1976, the Nurses' Health Study began. More than 120,000 nurses, ages 30 to 55, would be monitored to evaluate the effects of menopausal estrogen use on cardiovascular disease, cancers, and other health issues.

But the caution exhibited by doctors in prescribing hormones in the late 1970s was soon replaced by unfettered enthusiasm for the potential long-term health benefits of the drugs. The 1980s marked a time of scientific excitement and confusion about menopause hormones. In 1980, researchers showed that women who used estrogen had a 60 percent lower risk of hip fracture.[23] The first reports were published showing that women who used hormones had lower rates of cardiovascular disease and fewer heart attacks than women who didn't use hormone drugs.

Other studies showed that the risk of uterine cancer among hormone users could be reduced to a rate below that of non-hormone users if progestin was added to their treatment, the problem being that regular use of estrogen alone causes precancerous changes in the uterine lining. Adding progestin prevents thickening and other changes in the uterine lining triggered by estrogen, thereby reducing risk for uterine cancer.

While the benefits of progestin in terms of uterine cancer had been shown, little was known about the other effects progestin might have on a woman's health. Even so, doctors began prescribing it anyway. In response, Wyeth developed the drug Prempro, a combination of Premarin and the progestin medroxyprogesterone. Today, it's standard practice to prescribe a combination of estrogen and progestin for women who have a uterus. Women who have had a hysterectomy take only estrogen.

While the uterine cancer scare of 1975 had dampened enthusiasm for prescription hormones, the addition of progestin to the hormone mix reassured doctors and patients. Data showing a lower risk of cardiovascular disease and improved bone health among hormone users triggered a new wave of excitement about hormone therapy. While in the past, hormones had been thought of as a treatment to relieve menopause symptoms, doctors were beginning to believe that the potential was far greater — that hormones could give a boost to a woman's health by protecting her bones, her heart, and even her brain. The pendulum had swung again, and doctors stepped up their prescribing of hormones, whether or not a woman had menopause symptoms.

In 1990, Wyeth asked the FDA to approve the use of Premarin in women to prevent heart disease. The request was unusual because no controlled clinical trials had been conducted to prove whether there was a real benefit. Although an FDA advisory committee recommended approval, FDA officials pressed for more research.[24]

In an effort to learn more about the potential benefits of hormone therapy, the US government in 1991 began planning its largest-ever study of women's health, a massive undertaking that would come to be known as the Women's Health Initiative (WHI). The study prompted widespread debate in the medical community. Some researchers even believed such a study would be unethical, because women in the placebo group would be denied the benefits of hormone use.

By 2001, 42 percent of American women between ages 50 and 74 had used prescription hormones.[25] But by July 2002, the pendulum suddenly stopped completely. That's when officials from the NIH announced that they had halted the WHI hormone study.

3
HORMONES AND THE SYMPTOMS OF MENOPAUSE

The reason women decide to take menopause hormones is to relieve menopause symptoms. Sure, doctors still debate whether hormone use benefits women in other ways. But when a woman seeks out hormone treatment, she's not doing it because she's thinking about her long-term heart health. She's ripping the prescription out of her doctor's hand and racing to the pharmacy because she feels miserable and she wants to feel better.

If menopause was always easy, there wouldn't even be a hormone debate. The fact that women still want to know about hormones despite the controversy about heart attacks and breast cancer speaks volumes about the powerful and sometimes debilitating impact menopause has on a woman's life. To be sure, many women cope with the changes brought about by menopause just fine without any drug intervention. Other drug treatments and supplements also can help curb menopausal symptoms. But menopause hormones remain an important option because they are one of the most effective ways to treat some of the most frustrating symptoms associated with this life transition.

The decision about whether to take menopause hormones boils down to this: Will the benefits of these drugs for your personal health situation outweigh the small but real risks associated with using them? The first step in the hormone decision is to take an inventory of your symptoms and how they are affecting your life. It's a good idea to start a health diary to keep track of any health symptoms, mood changes, eating habits, and daily stressors. You can use a regular notebook or buy a special health diary at the bookstore. This will help you distinguish between symptoms that are minor annoyances and those that are truly disruptive to your life.

A health diary is also an important tool to help you look at the whole picture. For women today, midlife brings about many changes, not just menopause. Some of the health problems you might be attributing to menopause could be related to other issues. Caring for aging parents, having kids in high school or leaving for college, juggling work and family demands — all are factors contributing to your overall sense of well-being. By writing them down, you can begin to figure out the difference between menopausal symptoms and the general daily stress of being a woman.

To make sense of menopause, it helps to understand a little bit about the role your natural hormones have played so far, and what's happening inside your body as you make the menopausal transition.

A WOMAN'S OWN HORMONES

Menopause is not all bad. For roughly half of a woman's life, she has to deal with monthly periods, birth control, and the worries of an unwanted pregnancy. Menopause signals an end to all that — true freedom from the responsibilities of reproduction. That's a good thing, but getting there isn't always easy.

To understand what happens during menopause, it helps to learn a little about how hormones affect a woman's reproductive cycle. The defining female sex hormone is estrogen. It's responsible for breast development, periods, ovulation, and pregnancy. It influences blood pressure, cholesterol levels, bone health, cancer risk, and brain health.

When we think of a woman's natural estrogen, we typically are talking about estradiol. Estradiol is the main form of estrogen produced by the ovaries, and it's the dominant estrogen in the body prior to menopause. Estriol is the major estrogen produced during pregnancy. Estrone is the dominant form of estrogen found in your body after menopause.

Another important hormone is progesterone. Its main job is to get the body ready for pregnancy, and it's the dominant hormone during the second half of your menstrual cycle. (Progesterone is the hormone made by your body; progestin is the version of it made by drug companies.)

Estrogen and progesterone aren't the only hormones involved in the reproductive process. There's follicle-stimulating hormone (FSH) and luteinizing hormone (LH), which come from the pituitary gland. Other "releasing" hormones produced by the brain also play a role.

Here's how hormones work in the body to spur reproduction. FSH signals the ovaries to produce estrogen. Once estrogen levels reach a certain point, the brain tells the pituitary to shut down FSH and start making LH. LH spurs ovulation. Once an egg is

released, the ovaries start producing progesterone. This helps prepare the uterus for
conception. But if a woman doesn't get
pregnant — and most months she doesn't
— progesterone levels drop, and she gets
her period. This results in low levels of
estrogen and progesterone. The brain no-
tices that the hormones are low and sends a
signal that the body needs to step up FSH
production. Then the cycle starts all over
again.

So throughout life, hormone levels are
surging and falling to help spur the release
of eggs from a woman's ovaries and sustain
a pregnancy if needed. But a woman has
only so many eggs, and the ovaries can keep
releasing them for only so long. At some
point, usually about the fifth decade of a
woman's life, the ovaries start to shift gears.
They are heading to a life of semiretirement;
they will still be working but just not as
hard.

Like many transitions in life, it takes some
time for the body to work it out. When
estrogen levels are low, the brain orders up
a batch of FSH. If the ovaries are a bit slug-
gish and don't quickly respond with more
estrogen, the brain calls in more FSH. The
surge of FSH wakes up the ovaries and
prompts a burst of estrogen, sending a

woman's hormone levels far higher than normal for a little while. After working in overdrive, the ovaries slow down, and the body's hormone levels plunge.

Normally, this process is a result of natural aging. But there are some exceptions. Surgical menopause occurs when a woman has her ovaries removed. Losing her ovaries thrusts her into immediate menopause. Surgical menopause typically causes more severe symptoms than natural menopause. If the woman is very young at the time, hormone treatment is almost always recommended to help her body weather the stress of surgically induced menopause. Medical menopause is similar, in that drug treatments such as chemotherapy render the ovaries useless. And a small number of women experience menopause early in life for no obvious reason. This is called premature menopause.

PROBLEM PERIODS, BETTER SEX, AND THERMAL CHAOS

All the hormonal highs and lows associated with the menopausal transition create some subtle and not-so-subtle changes in a woman's body before, during, and after menopause. In the early part of the transition, a woman's period may not be as predictable.

It may be earlier or later than usual; there might be heavy bleeding or more light days than usual. Headaches and sleep problems may develop. Maintaining and losing weight may become more difficult as pounds start to accumulate around her middle.

And sex? Well, sex during these years can be an entirely different experience. Some women are more interested in sex than they've ever been, and everything about it just seems easier than in the past. Other women may notice that sometimes they're interested in sex, and other times they can't imagine ever wanting it again. Some women may lose interest entirely.

Here's a brief look at the various symptoms associated with menopause.

Hot flashes. The most-recognized symptom of menopause. Women who experience hot flashes feel flushed and warm. The sensation spreads throughout the body, leaving the woman soaked in sweat and then shivering with chills.

Night sweats. The nighttime version of the hot flash. All the same symptoms, except now you can't get back to sleep.

Sleep problems. Many women report changes in sleep patterns during menopause. Part of the problem may be night sweats that interrupt sleep. But changes in serotonin levels and other brain chemicals also likely result in sleep changes as we age.

Period changes. After menopause, a woman doesn't have periods anymore. But the menopausal transition can start a decade before actual menopause. For many women, this means irregular periods and heavy bleeding.

Headaches. Many women get headaches around the time of their periods. For some women, headaches triggered by fluctuating hormones are also part of menopause.

Mood swings. Remember PMS or the "baby blues"? Most women know that hormone changes from their periods and during and after pregnancy can have a big effect on their moods. So it's no surprise that menopause brings its own round of moodiness. Anxiety, irritability, crying jags, panic attacks, and depression may all be part of your menopausal experience.

Fuzzy thinking. Menopausal women often complain that their brains don't work the same way they once did. Fuzzy thinking, memory malfunctions, and concentration problems are typical complaints. Whether this is really menopause or just the stress of being a woman in midlife who doesn't get enough sleep remains a subject of debate. We'll discuss this further in Chapter 8.

Heart flutters. Many women report heart palpitations during menopause, often associated with hot flashes.

Vaginal dryness. Estrogen keeps vaginal tissue pliant and moisturized. As estrogen levels drop, the vagina shrinks and dries up. A woman may experience itching, burning, and painful sex due to lack of lubrication.

Urinary changes. Muscles that control urination lose their tone as estrogen levels drop. You may experience more-frequent urges to urinate; you may even find yourself waking up at night needing to pee. Urinary incontinence, when urine spills out before you're ready, also may develop.

Wrinkles. Natural estrogen plumps up your skin and keeps it elastic. Lower estrogen levels can lead to unwelcome changes in the appearance of your skin, causing it to sag and wrinkle.

Hair changes. Estrogen appears to affect hair quality. Some women report thinning and brittle hair after menopause. Others find that their hair gets straighter or curlier later in life.

Weight changes. Women in midlife tend to see their weight shift to their middles. How much this has to do with hormones isn't clear, although fluctuating hormone levels can affect appetite and spur eating binges in some women.

Fatigue. Fluctuating hormone levels, particularly low testosterone, may play a role in fatigue. Or it could be that you are just really busy and stressed out and not sleeping all that well.

Libido changes. Sex might be great, or it might be terrible. Or you might not be having it at all. Hormones certainly play a big role in this — but don't forget that how long you've been married, how much you like your partner, and how you feel about your body all influence your interest in sex.

Taking hormones in a pill will go a long way toward relieving many but not all of these symptoms. Some women may need only estrogen creams or vaginal rings. Others may find they need nothing at all. Which symptoms can be helped by hormones and which may be made worse will be discussed in future chapters. Other drug treatments also are available to relieve some of the symptoms of menopause; these will be discussed in Chapter 13.

UNDERSTANDING THE HOT FLASH

There are numerous symptoms associated with menopause, but for most women, the defining symptom is the hot flash. A hot flash is an uncomfortable wave of heat that moves through the body. Many people think it just leaves a woman red in the face, but during a hot flash, skin temperature and blood flow increase throughout the body. Studies show that skin temperature rises in the forehead, cheeks, upper arms, fingers, chest, abdomen, back, thighs, and calves. The woman starts to perspire as her body works hard to cool down. A hot flash can leave a woman drenched in sweat and shivering with chills simultaneously. Sometimes, hot flashes are accompanied by dizziness, heart palpitations, and feelings of severe anxiety or "suffocation."

In fact, the name "hot flash" doesn't do it justice. For many women, it's not some small flash of warmth but an overwhelming and debilitating experience.

Hot flashes are one of the main reasons women seek medical advice for menopause symptoms. Still, hot flashes remain a bit of a medical mystery. Even today, doctors know very little about why they happen and the best choices for treating them. In fact, the largest-ever study of menopause hormones — the Women's Health Initiative (WHI) — wasn't even designed to track hot flashes.

Hot and Bothered

Depending on what you read and whom you talk to, you'll hear various reports about how many women are affected by hot flashes. The Massachusetts Women's Health Study, one of the largest population-based studies of middle-aged women, has reported that about 75 percent of menopausal women experience hot flashes.[1] Among women who have hot flashes, most of them experience daily flashes that typically last 1 to 5 minutes.[2]

Your risk of suffering from hot flashes starts to increase during the 5 to 10 years prior to menopause. Hot flashes are at their worst and most frequent during the 2 years just after your last period; then they should start to decline. In one survey, about one-third of women between ages 35 and 47 began suffering from hot flashes before their periods even became irregular.[3]

For the purposes of consistency in research, the FDA has created definitions for mild, moderate, and severe hot flashes. A mild flash is a sensation of heat without sweating. A moderate flash is a sensation of heat with sweating, but the woman is able to continue doing whatever activity she is taking part in when the flash occurs. A severe flash is one that includes a sensation of heat and sweating so severe that the woman has to stop her activities to cope with and recover from the experience.[4]

A woman is considered to have only mild symptoms if she has fewer than seven hot flashes a day. As any woman would tell you, there is nothing mild about suffering sticky, heart-pounding flashes of heat, sweat, and chills seven times a day. Moderate to severe symptoms are defined as seven to eight moderate to severe flashes a day or 50 to 60 per week. About one-third of women who have hot flashes experience more than 10 a day.[5]

The real issue, of course, is how much of an impact hot flashes are having on your life. But knowing the definitions set forth by medical research can at least give you perspective in trying to determine how your symptoms stack up against other women's.

The good news is that hot flashes typically follow a consistent pattern in each woman. Once you realize that you are more likely to flash hourly or just weekly, you'll at least know what to expect. Hot flashes typically are at their worst in the early evening hours, when the body temperature peaks.

In the Study of Woman's Health Across the Nation (SWAN), researchers found that body weight may be one of the most important risk factors for hot flashes. Women with a body mass index above 27 were at higher risk for hot flashes than were thinner women.[6]

Hot flash rates also vary by ethnic group. In the SWAN study, hot flashes were reported by 45.6 percent of African American women, 35.4 percent of Hispanics, 31.2 percent of Caucasians, 20.5 percent of those of Chinese descent, and 17.6 percent of those of Japanese descent.[7] How long hot flashes will be part of your life also varies. One study found the average duration of hot flash symptoms among women to be 4 years. Another reported that two-thirds of menopausal women experience hot flashes for 1 to 5 years. The bottom line is that nobody knows if your flashes will last 6 months, 2 years, or 10 years. A small percentage of women continue to suffer hot flashes into their seventies.[8]

Are They All in Your Head?

Although the onset of hot flashes is linked with a woman's declining estrogen levels as she approaches menopause, hormones may not tell the whole story. It's becoming increasingly clear that hot flashes happen in the brain as well as the body.

Researchers at Wayne State University in

Detroit have dedicated their entire careers to understanding the hot flash. Recently, they studied a dozen menopausal women who were prone to hot flashes. To induce hot flashes, the researchers surrounded the women with heating pads. Then they took MRIs of the women's brains to try to determine what a brain looks like during a hot flash. They also compared the scans with those of women who weren't menopausal. The researchers saw significant changes in the part of the brain called the anterior insular cortex. This is the area where the body perceives sensations like temperature, pain, hunger, and erotic stimuli.

The scans support the theory that hot flashes are related to the body's ability to regulate its own temperature. The question is: What is it about menopause and declining estrogen levels that throws a woman's thermal regulation out of whack?

The Wayne State researchers have found that women who experience the most intense hot flashes are different from women who don't have hot flashes in how their bodies regulate temperature, sweating, and cooling down. Typically, the body regulates its core temperature in a neutral zone somewhere between an upper limit for sweating and a lower limit for shivering. In measuring the different points when women start to perspire, the researchers have shown that women who suffer from hot flashes don't really have this neutral zone.

The neutral zone that helps regulate body temperature appears to be influenced by norepinephrine, a stress hormone that pumps you up in times of crisis. Norepinephrine could explain the heart pounding that accompanies a hot flash. It also may act on the hypothalamus, the part of the brain that regulates the body's thermostat. Although it's not clear why, a woman's declining estrogen levels may send a message to the brain triggering a release of norepinephrine, playing a role in the cascade of events that culminates in a hot flash. In animal experiments, increased brain norepinephrine narrows the thermoneutral zone.

We've known for a long time that taking estrogen in a pill helps curb hot flashes, but we didn't always know why. It may be that taking estrogen widens the thermoneutral zone in women, allowing their bodies to better regulate core body temperature and reducing the chance that they will suffer a hot flash. To figure this out, the Wayne State researchers have studied how the body regulates temperature in women who take hormones compared with those who do not. After both groups of women were wrapped in heating pads, the researchers measured how quickly they started sweating. Women taking hormone drugs stayed cool longer, meaning they started sweating later than the nonusers did. This suggests that menopause hormones aren't curbing hot flashes simply by replacing estrogen. The hormones appear to act on the brain in a way that raises the sweating threshold and makes a woman less vulnerable to the thermal fluctuations associated with menopause.

This knowledge is beginning to help us understand why certain drugs and treatments help relieve hot flashes. But the bottom line is that core-body temperature regulation plays an important role in hot flash risk. Yes, your hormones are calling the shots, but staying cool, wearing light layers of clothing, drinking lots of cold beverages, and air-conditioning your environment can all help avert hot flashes. Weight loss can also help because it reduces the amount of body fat "insulation."

DOES TAKING HORMONES JUST DELAY THE INEVITABLE?

The fact that hormones sometimes only delay symptoms, rather than stopping them, is the dirty little secret of the menopause hormone business. For many women, taking hormones in a pill will ease their symptoms and make menopause a whole lot easier to get through. Ideally, a woman will take the hormones only during this time to smooth out the volatile hormonal fluctuations going on inside her body. Eventually, the theory goes, her body will calm down, and she won't need the hormones any more. The plan is for hormones in a pill to essentially work as a bridge to get a woman through the worst part of menopause. Unfortunately, it doesn't always work that way.

First, there is a small percentage of women who will always have menopausal symptoms if they don't take hormones or other treatments. One Swedish study reported that 9 percent of women at age 72 were still suffering from hot flashes. There's no way to know now whether you are one of these women.

Second, if you are taking hormones, it's impossible to know how long your own symptoms would last if you weren't taking them, so it's hard to gauge when is a good time to stop. It's all pretty much guesswork. If you try to stop the hormones after about 2 years, and your symptoms come back with a vengeance, then your doctor might suggest taking the pills for another year or two. The FDA says that women should take hormones in the lowest dose for the shortest possible duration for the relief of symptoms. Nobody really knows what that means, but most doctors interpret it as no more than 4 to 5 years, and less if possible.

This is where it gets tricky. Your body becomes accustomed to the extra hormones you're giving it. When you decide to stop the pills, there's a chance you will go through some version of withdrawal, and you may develop "rebound" symptoms. These are caused not by the natural hormonal conditions of your body but by the drugs you've been taking to prevent the symptoms in the first place. There's not a lot of research on this rebound effect. Quitting cold turkey is probably a bad idea; most doctors suggest slowly weaning off the drugs to ease your body into a life without hormones.

Most women will do fine as they taper off hormones. But some will start to have symptoms again, and the symptoms may be more severe than when the women first started using the drugs. We now have a fair amount of data on this as a result of the WHI. Not only were women in the study told to stop taking their pills literally overnight, but after the results were announced, scores of other women stopped the drugs cold turkey as well.

The medical journal *Maturitas* tracked 205 women who had used hormones for an average of 4 years but quit immediately after the WHI findings became public. The good news is that 56 percent of the women didn't have hot flashes or other so-called vasomotor symptoms after quitting the drugs. But that means 44 percent did continue to have symptoms, although it's not clear from the study how long the symptoms lasted. Only about 5 percent of the women had mood problems, while 11 percent had multiple symptoms.[9]

The most interesting data on quitting hormones came from the WHI. The researchers followed up with these women, including more than 900 who had moderate or severe hot flashes when the study began. The research represents the best data we have to date on the effects of stopping hormones.

Among women who had symptoms at the start of the study, those who took hormones were more likely than those in the placebo group to still have symptoms after stopping the pills.[10] This may suggest that hormone users were experiencing a rebound effect from the drugs. Or it could mean that women in the placebo group completed the menopausal transition during the study period, while women who were taking the hormones simply delayed it. Some data suggest that the return of symptoms is brief, peaking at about 8 weeks after stopping treatment.

Knowing that the symptoms might return after stopping hormone drugs is certainly an issue you should factor into your overall hormone decision. For some women, taking hormones still might make sense. Many women are helped by hormones and find it easy to transition off the drugs without experiencing a return of symptoms. Even if you are going to have to deal with menopause symptoms eventually, you may have a lot of good reasons to want to delay the experience. If you are raising kids or working in a demanding job, it may be that you just don't have time for menopause right now.

THE NEXT STEP

Keep a health diary and track your symptoms. Make a list of the symptoms that are particularly disruptive or troublesome. This is the starting point for your hormone decision. Now keep reading to learn about the various risks and benefits of hormones.

■ ■ ■ ■

PART TWO:
UNDERSTANDING THE
SCIENCE

■ ■ ■ ■

4
HORMONES AND
YOUR HEART

Right now, you are probably more concerned about hot flashes and getting a good night's sleep than you are about your heart. But every menopausal woman — whether or not she chooses to use hormones — needs to think about her heart health. Cardiovascular disease — which leads to heart attack and stroke — kills more than 500,000 women a year, making it the greatest threat to women's health. That means that 1 in 2 female deaths are from heart disease or stroke, compared with 1 in 25 women who will eventually die of breast cancer.[1]

Heart disease is characterized by a narrowing of the arteries that lead to the heart. This process, called atherosclerosis, is caused by the buildup of cholesterol and fat into plaques, which are hardened deposits on the artery walls. If an artery becomes clogged — either by a blood clot or by a piece of floating plaque — the woman has a heart attack. The process can also occur in the arteries that supply blood to the brain, resulting in stroke.

Granted, we are all going to die of something someday, and everyone's heart wears out eventually. Heart disease risk jumps when a woman turns 50, but most women don't start having heart attacks until they're in their seventies. (The average age for a first heart attack for a woman is 74.[2]) But menopause is an important milestone for a woman's heart. At the time of menopause, women undergo many changes that affect their cardiovascular health. Hopefully, you've already adopted the lifestyle changes like a healthful diet, exercise, and stress management that will help your heart stay young. If you haven't, it's not too late to start.

The effect of hormones — the kind made by our bodies and the kind made by drug companies — on the heart is a matter of heated medical and scientific debate. Many women today have the perception that hormones cause heart attacks, based on the headlines generated by the release of data from the Women's Health Initiative (WHI). But more-recent analyses of the data show that simply isn't the case for the typical hormone user. For the average woman considering hormones to treat the symptoms of menopause, the data from the WHI are actually reassuring. There weren't a lot of younger menopausal women participating in the WHI, but what little data we have show that the benefits of hormones for these women likely outweigh the risks.

While the medical community was initially shocked by the results of the WHI, a closer look at the data shows that the latest hormone research is surprisingly consistent with earlier studies of hormones and heart health. Some of those other studies have suggested that hormones protect a woman from heart disease, some have shown no benefit, and some have suggested that hormones may increase risk for heart troubles in certain women. All three of these trends have shown up in the WHI data.

Although science is beginning to make sense of much of the hormone data, there is still one major point of contention among scientists — that is, whether hormones might provide added heart protection for some women. According to some research, this may in fact be the case.

Let's be perfectly clear here: Most doctors don't recommend that a woman take hormones in the hope of boosting her heart health. There simply isn't enough evidence to justify hormone use to protect your heart, and there are other, far more effective and proven ways to stay heart healthy. For example, a large body of evidence suggests that lifestyle changes like eating a balanced diet, getting regular exercise, controlling blood pressure, lowering cholesterol, preventing and managing diabetes, and possibly even taking a daily low-dose aspirin do a better job of preventing heart disease than using hormones does.

So why even talk about the possibility of hormones offering extra heart protection? Because doctors and scientists are talking about it, and you're likely to hear conflicting information related to hormones and heart risk.

Some doctors still firmly believe that there is a benefit to the heart from starting hormones at menopause and taking them for the rest of your life. After reading more about the early studies of hormones and heart health, you'll understand why so many experts still believe there might be something to this theory. Others will argue that heart disease risk is reason enough not to take hormones. Purveyors of so-called "bio-identical hormones" often cite WHI data to support switching to these pharmacy-mixed hormones. (We'll talk about this in Chapter 13.)

But the people at the extremes of the debate over hormones and heart health — those who say that hormones are definitely good for your heart or obviously bad for your heart — simply aren't paying attention to the science. For you to distinguish between the facts and the hype, you need a full understanding of what science shows us about how hormones affect women's hearts. We don't have all the answers, but we are getting closer.

THE MENOPAUSAL HEART

Doctors have long speculated that a woman's natural estrogen protects her heart. One of the main reasons for this is that a woman's risk of heart attack doesn't start to increase until she's past 50. This is a full decade later than the age at which men first start having heart attacks. Estrogen isn't the only difference between men and women, but it is an obvious and important one.

One reason scientists have focused on estrogen is that surgical menopause (removing a woman's ovaries) seems to be associated with a markedly increased risk of heart trouble. In 1959, scientists first noticed that women who had their ovaries removed were at higher risk for heart problems.[3] Later, doctors realized that if they replaced the estrogen lost as a result of the surgery with estrogen drugs, the higher heart disease risk disappeared. This finding sent scientists in pursuit of estrogen as the explanation for why women's hearts stay healthy longer than men's hearts.

So convinced were scientists that estrogen offered added heart protection that they even tried treating men with it. In the 1970s, the Coronary Drug Project gave two groups of men with known heart disease different doses of Premarin. But the study was stopped because the men who took estrogen developed higher rates of blood clots and heart attacks.[4]

Estrogen probably doesn't explain all the differences between men's and women's hearts. While the loss of natural estrogen may be part of the reason women are at higher risk for heart attack after menopause, it also may be that menopause simply coincides with other changes in a woman's body due to aging. At menopause, for example, a woman will notice changes in her blood cholesterol levels. Total and LDL cholesterol — the bad kind of cholesterol that should stay low — starts to rise. HDL cholesterol, the good cholesterol that should be high, starts to decline. Fibrinogen, a substance in the blood that can increase the risk of clotting, also starts to rise.[5]

THE FIRST HORMONE AND HEART STUDIES

In 1985, two hormone studies that seemed to directly contradict each other were published at the same time. The first was the Framingham Heart Study, a well-respected study started in 1948 that tracked the health of 5,209 men and women from the town of Framingham, Massachusetts. The study showed that among 1,234 women over an 8-year period, those who used estrogen had nearly twice the risk of cardio-vascular disease.[6] But the finding was confusing because it became public at the same time as a report from the Nurses' Health Study, another highly regarded Harvard study. It showed that among more than 32,000 nurses, those who used estrogen were 50 percent less likely to experience a heart attack.[7]

It's not clear why two similar studies produced such conflicting results, but the incongruity was soon forgotten as other observational research showed hormones to be protective, supporting the findings of the Nurses' Health Study. In 1987, the Lipid Research Clinics Follow-Up suggested that estrogen boosted heart health by raising HDL cholesterol. In that study, 2,270 women between ages 40 and 69 were followed for more than 8 years, during which time estrogen users showed a 63 percent lower risk of heart attack.[8] A year later, a study by Kaiser Permanente California of more than 6,000 women linked estrogen use with fewer heart attacks.[9]

By 1991, it seemed virtually certain that taking estrogen at menopause helped lower a woman's risk of heart attack. A second report from the Nurses' Health Study showed that among nearly 50,000 nurses, estrogen users had a 44 percent lower risk of heart disease than nonusers.[10] That was followed by a landmark review of all the observational studies to date evaluating hormones and heart health. This was a meta-analysis, meaning it used sophisticated statistical techniques to combine the data from all the studies. It showed that study participants who used estrogen had cut their overall risk of heart problems by at least one-third.[11]

Most of the women tracked in these early observational studies were using only estrogen. But a handful of studies suggested that women also could benefit if they were taking a combination of estrogen and progestin. In a review of seven studies involving women taking both estrogen and progestin, hormone users still showed a 34 percent lower risk of heart problems than non-users.[12]

Reviewing this research, even today, makes a pretty convincing case that hormones seem to have something to do with the health of a woman's heart. But a pressing question remains: Were hormones keeping these women healthy? Or was it simply that healthy women were choosing hormones?

All the data on the benefits of menopause hormones had so far come from observational studies, which track the health habits of study participants over time. An observational study can show trends, but it can't answer specific questions. Further, the women in the studies make their own choices about whether or not to take hormones. In all the observational studies, women who took estrogen after menopause were more likely to be white, educated, upper-middle class, and lean — all factors associated with a lower risk of heart disease.[13] So did hormones protect the heart? Did education protect the heart? Or did being lean protect the heart? Nobody knew exactly what role hormones were playing in the heart health of these women.

With such overwhelming evidence from the observational studies, it was time to try to find out why hormone users seemed to have healthier hearts. The real test of hormones would come from clinical trials, in which women don't choose their own treatments but instead are randomly selected to receive either hormones or a placebo.

One of the first projects was the 1995 Postmenopausal Estrogen/Progestin Interventions, or the PEPI trial. The women in the trial — all between ages 45 and 65 — took estrogen alone, a combined estrogen/progestin regimen, or a placebo. The PEPI study showed that hormones boosted good cholesterol and lowered bad cholesterol. Adding progestin slightly dampened the impact on HDL, but overall, hormones seemed to improve a woman's cholesterol profile.[14]

While PEPI identified one way in which hormones might help women's hearts — by lowering bad cholesterol and raising good cholesterol — it didn't tell us if those changes made any real difference to women's health. The thinking at the time was that because hormones appeared to help women's hearts, they should be given to women at highest risk for heart problems —

108

those with established heart disease or a history of heart attack.

As a result, the drugmaker Wyeth, which sells Premarin and Prempro, paid for the first large clinical trial to examine whether hormones affect a woman's risk of heart attack. The Heart and Estrogen/Progestin Replacement Study (HERS) was disappointing. Nearly 2,800 women with documented heart disease were given either estrogen plus progestin or a placebo for about 4 years. The average age of the women in the study was 67 years. The women who took hormones showed big drops in bad cholesterol and big jumps in good cholesterol, but there was no difference in the rate of heart attack between the hormone users and nonusers. Most notable was the fact that the hormone users had a 50 percent higher risk of heart problems during the first year of treatment.[15]

The HERS and some subsequent trials of hormones in women with heart problems made it clear that estrogen therapy wasn't appropriate for older women who already had heart disease. But this didn't rule out the possibility that estrogen could benefit the hearts of younger women. It simply showed that once heart disease sets in, it's too late for estrogen to make a difference.

Estrogen clearly doesn't repair the damage from heart disease, but the question remains as to whether estrogen helps protect a healthy young woman from developing heart disease in the first place.

MONKEY HEARTS AND HORMONES

You may not think you have much in common with a monkey, but you do — 94 percent of your DNA, to be exact. Some of the most provocative research suggesting that the timing of hormone therapy makes a difference in its effects on heart health comes from studies of menopausal monkeys at the Wake Forest University School of Medicine in Winston-Salem, North Carolina. The study doesn't yield any definitive conclusions about how hormones affect women — it did involve monkeys, after all — but it does give us some important clues.

The Wake Forest researchers induced menopause in cynomolgus macaques by removing their ovaries. After the surgical menopause procedure, some of the monkeys were given Prempro, the drug that combines estrogen and progestin, while some of the monkeys didn't take any hormones. All were fed heart-disease-inducing diets consisting of lard, butter, and eggs. After 3 years, the monkeys on hormones had up to 70 percent less plaque buildup in their arteries than the monkeys that were not given hormones.

More interesting was a third group of monkeys. They had their ovaries removed at the same time as the other animals, but they weren't given hormones for 2 years after the procedure. In the third year, they started receiving Prempro. That 2-year delay in monkey years is the equivalent of a woman waiting 6 years after menopause to begin hormone therapy. While hormones started immediately prevented plaque buildup in one group of monkeys, the monkeys whose hormone treatment was delayed had about the same level of plaque as those that didn't receive hormones at all. The study suggests that Prempro preserves artery health when started early, but it can't repair the damage once heart disease sets in.

THE WOMEN'S HEALTH INITIATIVE: DOES TIMING OF HORMONE USE REALLY MATTER?

Whether estrogen helped the hearts of healthy women was exactly the question the WHI was supposed to answer. But for the reasons I explained in Chapter 1, that's not the study we ended up with. It would take years for young menopausal women to become old enough to start having heart attacks. As a result, the investigators decided that the only way to measure the impact of hormones on heart health in the time allotted for the WHI was to choose older women for the study. So instead of being a study of young healthy women, the WHI looked at menopause hormone use in mostly older women long past menopause.

Of the 27,000 women participating in the WHI hormone trials, only 3,425 were under age 55. The average age of the women in the WHI was 63, not much younger than the average 67-year-old in the HERS investigation. Most women in the WHI started hormones at least 10 years past menopause. By comparison, the women in the Nurses' Health Study — which showed that hormones lowered heart attack risk by as much as 50 percent — were between ages 30 and 55 when they started using hormones for either surgical or natural menopause. Further, 90 percent of the women in the nurses' study started hormones within 4 years of the onset of menopause.

But women are women, aren't they? Does the age of the women really matter? Is there really that much difference between a 53-year-old woman, a 63-year-old, and a 73-year-old? Subsequent age breakdowns of the WHI data show that age probably does matter when it comes to the risks and benefits of hormones. Even more important than age seems to be is the *timing* of hormone use relative to menopause. What we know now is that the women in the WHI who started hormones during or less than 10 years after menopause did far better than the women who started hormones 10 years or more after menopause.

ESTROGEN, PROGESTIN, AND THE HEART

Let's explore the broad conclusions about hormones and heart risk that were drawn from the WHI and how the results shift when women are studied by age group and time since menopause.

First, let's look at the group of women who took Prempro, the combination of estrogen and progestin. Overall, the women in the WHI were tracked for an average of 5.2 years. Those who used Prempro had a 24 percent higher risk of heart attack. The highest risk came in the first year, with an 81 percent increase in risk. After that, risk tapered off. Among those women tracked for 6 years or more, hormone use actually resulted in a 30 percent reduction in heart problems by the sixth year.

Don't be too alarmed by these numbers. For most menopausal women, the risk of having a heart attack is very low to start with, so a 24 percent increase in risk still translates to a very low risk overall. It means that among 10,000 women, 30 would have heart problems due to normal aging. Among 10,000 women taking estrogen and progestin, 37 would have heart problems — meaning the hormones raised risk for 7 of 10,000 women.[16] But again, given the large number of older women in the WHI, even these numbers probably don't apply to most women who are considering menopause hormones.

Before we continue, it's important to note that little of the heart and hormone data from the WHI reached the point of statistical significance. This is a critical scientific threshold that helps researchers determine if the trends they've identified are real and directly related to the treatment involved or are simply due to chance. As I explained in Chapter 1, the lack of statistical significance of much of the WHI data has made interpreting the research very frustrating. The National Institutes of Health has been largely inconsistent about what trends from the WHI they single out as being important for women's health and what trends they readily dismiss. Unfortunately, this is the only data we have, and we need to make the best of it.

Even though many of the findings from the WHI didn't reach statistical significance, they shouldn't be ignored, especially since they're from such a large and important study. For instance, the overall finding that the Prempro users had a 24 percent higher risk of heart attack just missed statistical significance by the narrowest of margins. The finding of highest risk in the first year is scientifically valid. Unfortunately, none of the other data from the Prempro study looking at risk of heart attack by age, time since menopause, or health status is statistically meaningful.

So how do we know if the trends are real? Much of the data from the WHI has been compared with data from other clinical trials and observational studies, and the trends are consistent across studies among women of similar ages. While we can't always draw definitive conclusions from much of the WHI data, paying attention to it certainly makes sense when we are trying to weigh all the risks and benefits of hormone use. So we know that overall, in this study of mostly older women who started hormones long past menopause, hormone use increased risk of heart attack by 24 percent over 5 years and 81 percent in the first year.

Now let's look at women in the estrogen/

progestin segment of the WHI who started hormones within 10 years of menopause. They actually had an 11 percent *lower* risk of heart problems. By comparison, women in the WHI who started hormones 10 years after menopause had a 22 percent *higher* risk of heart attack. As surprising as it is, the WHI included many women who started taking hormones 20 years past menopause. Those women had a 71 percent higher risk of heart attack than non-hormone users 20 years past menopause.[17]

Other data from this segment of the WHI also support the idea that hormone therapy initiated at the time of menopause is safe compared with hormone therapy started long after menopause. Consider the women in the 50 to 59 age group. Overall, these women still had a 27 percent higher risk of heart problems if they used hormones. Based on this statistic alone, hormone therapy may seem no safer for younger women than for older women. What we need to keep in mind is that in the WHI, even the younger women were several years past menopause. This is why researchers decided to compare the women in the 50 to 59 age group who were having hot flashes with those who weren't. A hot flash is a pretty good sign that your body is still experiencing the hormonal fluctuations associated with the menopausal transition. Young women with hot flashes had a 5 percent lower risk of heart problems. Young women who no longer had hot flashes — suggesting they were long past menopause — had a stunning 98 percent higher risk of heart troubles.[18]

Because these data aren't statistically sound, women shouldn't conclude from it that hormones taken close to menopause will protect their hearts. However, these data should offer important reassurance that hormone therapy initiated close to menopause to treat menopause symptoms won't increase a woman's risk of heart attack.

ESTROGEN ALONE AND THE HEART

Women who have undergone a hysterectomy and who take estrogen by itself have been unnecessarily frightened by the WHI data. The original WHI study of estrogen and progestin was stopped early because of worries about heart attacks and breast cancer. However, there was no overall elevated heart risk among the women in the WHI who took estrogen alone. In fact, women who used estrogen alone had 5 percent fewer heart problems than nonusers.[19] Like other parts of the WHI, little of the data about estrogen therapy and heart health is statistically meaningful.

The breakdown of women who use estrogen alone, by age and time since menopause, again paints a reassuring picture. Women between ages 50 and 59 who used estrogen had a 37 percent lower risk of heart attack compared with women who received a placebo. The apparent benefits of estrogen use dropped to just 6 percent in the 60 to 69 age group. And 70- to 79-year-old estrogen users had an 11 percent *higher* risk of heart problems than nonusers in the same age group. The clear picture is that estrogen use started at the time of surgical or natural menopause is safe for the heart and may even offer some protection. But waiting long past menopause to take estrogen is risky.

COMPARING THE WHI AND THE NURSES' HEALTH STUDY

Some of the most important scientific research of menopause hormones to emerge in recent years hasn't gotten much attention. Researchers have taken the data from the WHI and tried to compare it with the important data generated by the famous Nurses' Health Study — the first major study to suggest that hormones may offer added protection to women's hearts. The problem with comparing the two studies is that the study populations were so different. In general, the women in the nurses' study started hormone therapy at a young age, and the majority used estrogen alone. In the WHI, most of the women started hormones at an older age, long past menopause, and the majority used a combination of estrogen and progestin.

Yet there is some overlap between the two studies. What is so important about this comparison is that it shows that the WHI results weren't as shocking as they first seemed to be. In fact, the WHI data are remarkably consistent with much of the observational study data and other clinical trial data that came before it. Again, the biggest problem with the WHI was the scaremongering fashion in which the data were presented to the public. The data alone aren't that scary.

Both the WHI and the Nurses' Health Study report virtually identical increases in risk of stroke and blood clots among hormone users, compared with the risk among nonusers. But the studies seem to paint markedly different pictures of heart attack risk from hormone use. The Nurses' Health Study has shown that women who took hormones were 40 to 50 percent less likely to suffer heart attacks than nonusers. But the WHI estrogen and progestin study concluded that hormone use increases a woman's heart attack risk by 24 percent. The WHI estrogen-only study showed that there was no overall benefit or risk to the heart related to hormone use.

But let's take a look at the nurses who most closely resembled the women in the WHI. These nurses started hormone therapy at least 10 years after menopause. In this group, hormones offered little, if any, heart protection. These women had up to a 31 percent higher relative risk of heart attack than the nurses who started hormones close to menopause. Notably, this is similar to the women in the WHI who started hormones 10 or more years past menopause. They had a 37 percent higher relative risk of heart attack compared with those in the study who started hormone therapy sooner.

A comparison of both studies suggests that women who start hormones close to menopause appear to lower their risk of heart attack. The nurses who started hormones within 4 years of menopause had up to a 34 percent lower risk of heart attack than nonusers. Women in the WHI who started hormones within 10 years of menopause had an 11 percent lower risk.[20]

OTHER HEART HEALTH FACTORS TO CONSIDER

In addition to questions raised about the timing of hormone therapy, the WHI data raise concerns about certain heart-related health factors that may contribute to the risks and benefits of hormones. These aren't well researched yet, but since they are trends that emerged in the WHI, they are worth considering in the context of your hormone decision.

Cholesterol. Both the estrogen/progestin and estrogen-alone studies suggested that the risks and benefits of hormones change depending on a woman's overall cholesterol level. We already know that high cholesterol can be a risk factor for heart disease. But the WHI data show that combining high cholesterol with hormone use further increases the risk of heart problems. Conversely, low cholesterol combined with hormone use seems to further reduce risk of heart problems.

In the estrogen/progestin study, among women whose total cholesterol exceeded 242 mg/dl (milligrams per deciliter of blood), hormone users had a two-fold increase in heart attack risk. Among women whose total cholesterol was lower than 208 mg/dl, hormone use was associated with a 24 percent *reduction* in heart attack risk. These trends held up when looking at bad cholesterol and good cholesterol. Among hormone users, LDL cholesterol of more than 155 mg/dl correlated to a 68 percent increase in heart attack risk, while LDL cholesterol below 126 mg/dl correlated to a 14 percent reduction in heart attack risk. As for HDL cholesterol, women with HDL levels below 47 mg/dl had an 86 percent higher risk of heart problems if they also used hormones. By comparison, hormone users with HDL levels exceeding 58 mg/dl were 12 percent less likely to suffer heart attacks.[21]

The trends were less pronounced but similar among women taking estrogen alone. For those with low LDL and high HDL, estrogen use resulted in further reductions in heart attack risk. On the other hand, a high level of bad cholesterol and not enough good cholesterol meant a higher heart attack risk among hormone users compared with non-hormone users.[22]

So what does this mean for you? The data aren't statistically meaningful, so we have to be careful not to overstate their importance.

However, we already know that high total cholesterol, high LDL, and low HDL are associated with a higher heart disease risk. We also know from other studies that women with established heart disease should not take hormones because hormone use actually increases risk if you already are prone to heart troubles. So if you are a woman with poor cholesterol scores, you should consider your overall heart health when making the decision whether to use hormones.

The good news is that a class of drugs called statins is highly effective in lowering cholesterol. Both WHI hormone studies showed that woman who took statins at the time they joined the study (suggesting they had high cholesterol that was being treated) didn't have any higher risk of heart problems when using hormones.

Blood pressure/diabetes. Women in the estrogen/progestin studies with high blood pressure or diabetes had double the heart attack risk of women without these health problems. In the estrogen-only group, having diabetes or high blood pressure didn't make any difference in overall risk.

Body mass index/waist circumference. In the estrogen-only group, having a lower body mass index and lower waist circumference further reduced heart attack risk. Women with a body mass index below 25 and a waist circumference below 85 centimeters (about 33.5 inches) showed a 22 to 24 percent reduction in heart attack risk compared with similar-size women who were not taking estrogen. But women who were obese, with waist sizes that exceeded 38 inches, were at slightly higher risk for heart problems if they were using hormones compared with similar-size women who weren't using the drugs. Again, both waist circumference and body mass index are indicators of overall health and risk for heart problems. So a woman who is overweight or who has a thick waist needs to pay extra attention to her health as she ages.

The conclusions you should draw from this are obvious. The healthier you are before you start taking hormones, the healthier you will be while you are on hormones. The risks and benefits of these drugs seem to be enhanced or worsened depending on the overall health of the woman who uses them. Most important, analyses of data from the WHI and the Nurses' Health Study show that the differences in health risks and benefits seen among hormone users disappear when the women follow a healthful diet and get regular exercise. That means if you are eating right and staying physically active, you simply don't have to worry about how hormones may affect your heart. You already are doing everything you should to lower your heart disease risk.

LOOKING AHEAD

A closer examination of the WHI data has given us reassuring information about the safety of hormones for women who want to use them to treat the symptoms of menopause. Though older women long past menopause should not use hormones, those who are undergoing surgical menopause or experiencing the symptoms of natural menopause can take comfort in the knowledge that choosing hormones does not put their hearts at risk.

However, not everybody is satisfied. Many people still believe that women will benefit from starting hormones at menopause and staying on them indefinitely. Others simply want more definitive information about the health impact of hormones in women who use them for menopause symptoms because the WHI data really aren't statistically reliable.

As a result, an important study called KEEPS is under way. KEEPS, which stands for Kronos Early Estrogen and Progestin Study, is funded by billionaire John Sperling. Sperling owns the Kronos Optimal Health Centre, a clinic in Scottsdale, Arizona. Doctors at Kronos routinely prescribe hormone therapy to menopausal women. Mr. Sperling has long believed that regular doses of the right medicine can keep people healthy well into old age.

Sperling and the doctors at Kronos, like many doctors around the world, were upset with the way the WHI results were released and the broad conclusions that have been drawn from them. As a result, Sperling kicked in $14 million of his own money to fund a trial that will evaluate hormone use in women at the time of menopause.[23] The study isn't big enough or long enough to measure heart attack risk. However, it hopes to do the next best thing by using various tests to measure early indicators of heart disease, such as the thickness of the carotid artery in the neck and the amount of calcium in the coronary arteries. The data won't be conclusive, but they will certainly supply some important pieces for the hormone puzzle. Notably, some of the top doctors involved in the WHI heart research also will take part in the KEEPS trial.

5
HORMONES AND
YOUR BREASTS

There is no question that hormones influence a woman's chances of developing breast cancer. But it's not just the hormones that she may be taking to help cope with menopause symptoms. The hormones in birth control pills, and even the hormones produced by the body, influence breast cancer risk to some extent throughout a woman's life. Scientists are still trying to figure out how much risk these various hormone exposures pose to women during their lifetimes, but the full effect of hormones on breast cancer remains puzzling.

The most recent hormone research has further complicated the picture, showing that there may be two very different breast cancer stories for menopausal women using hormones. First, women who use a combination of estrogen and progestin appear to have a slightly higher risk of breast cancer than women who don't use hormones. The risk isn't enormous, and it has to be weighed against the other risks and benefits of hormone drugs. The good news is that recent studies have finally given us detailed information about the time frame during which menopause hormones are likely to be safest for women's breasts. And there are steps women can take to further lower the risk of using hormones to treat menopause symptoms.

The second and perhaps more surprising story involves women who use only estrogen. These are women who have had a hysterectomy, so they don't need to worry about uterine cancer, which is cancer of the uterine lining, or endometrium. (A woman who still has her uterus takes both estrogen and progestin, which protects against uterine cancer. But if you've had your uterus removed in a hysterectomy, you don't need progestin.) Recent studies show that women who have undergone a hysterectomy and use estrogen by itself during menopause may get some added protection against breast cancer. The idea that estrogen therapy may protect a woman from breast cancer has created a great deal of excitement among medical researchers. Not everyone is convinced that there is a benefit, or even that there's no harm from taking estrogen alone. Nonetheless, this research is reassuring to many women — even as it has raised further questions about the role of estrogen as well as progestin in breast cancer.

To make sense of all this, let's begin by exploring what science has shown us over the years about the relationship between hormones — those made by a woman's body and those from outside sources like pills and patches — and breast cancer. *An important note of caution:* As you read through this information, some of the statistics may seem frightening. Various studies have found a range of increased risks associated with hormone use, and when given as percentages, they sound big and scary. But it's important to remember that even a large percentage increase in risk typically translates into only a slight change in overall risk.

In general, the risk of developing breast cancer increases with age. Rates are generally low in women under 40, start to increase after 40, and are highest in those 70 and older. The average age of breast cancer diagnosis is 62.

At the end of this chapter, I will give you some tools that will help you understand your risk of breast cancer currently and over the next 5 to 30 years, based on your personal health history and lifestyle. Once you know your existing risk of breast cancer, these tools will help you better assess how much of an increase in risk — if any — you will experience if you choose to take meno-pause hormones.

HORMONES FROM WITHIN

The hormones estrogen and progesterone are in many ways the essence of woman-hood. They are essential to the function of a woman's ovaries and to her ability to repro-duce and prepare the womb to incubate a baby. They are the "sex hormones" that distinguish a woman's body from a man's, influencing breast development, mood, desire, and possibly even a woman's cardio-vascular health and longevity. Knowing this, it's difficult to understand why a woman's exposure to her own hormones can also af-fect her risk of breast cancer. But numerous scientific studies show that a woman's *en-dogenous* hormones — those made by her body — are part of a complex equation of both enhancing health and detracting from it.

One of the first signs that a woman's own hormones are linked to breast cancer came in a 1968 report in the *Journal of the National Cancer Institute.* This study looked at artificial menopause, which occurs when a woman undergoes surgical removal of her ovaries or receives radiation or other treatments that stop the ovaries' natural function. The researchers studied more than 9,000 women who had experienced artificial menopause and compared them with women experiencing natural menopause. The women who had their ovaries and uterus removed before age 40 were 75 percent less likely to develop breast cancer than women who kept their ovaries. This suggested that lifetime exposure to ovarian hormones likely played a role in a woman's risk of breast cancer.[1]

Since those early studies, scientific data have continued to support the idea that a woman's exposure to her own hormones influences her chances of developing breast cancer. Many of these findings are from the Nurses' Health Study, the ongoing study by Harvard researchers that has tracked the health and lifestyle habits of more than 120,000 nurses since 1976. Women who started menstruating at an early age (before 12) or who went through menopause at a late age (after 55) have a slightly higher risk of breast cancer. So that means the later you start your period and the earlier you enter menopause, the less likely you are to develop breast cancer.

Having a baby before age 30 also lowers a woman's risk of breast cancer. So, too, may breastfeeding for a year or more, according to some studies. What's the common denominator here? It may be that pregnancy and breastfeeding reduce a woman's lifetime number of menstrual cycles. The later you start your period and the earlier you reach menopause also reduce the number of menstrual cycles your body experiences — and that, in turn, lowers the cumulative exposure of your breasts to estrogen and other sex hormones.

One effect of high natural estrogen levels is that a woman is more likely to have stronger bones and denser breast tissue. Women with dense breasts and dense bones are known to be slightly more likely to develop breast cancer — another indicator that high natural estrogen levels influence breast cancer risk.

Beyond deciding when to have a baby and whether to breastfeed, a woman really doesn't have much control over the factors that determine her exposure to her body's own estrogens. There is one other way in which she can limit her exposure: by maintaining a healthy weight. Body fat is essentially a source of estrogen, and women who have more body fat usually have more of their own estrogen than women who are thin. The Nurses' Health Study taught us that among postmenopausal women, obesity is associated with higher levels of estrogen and an increased risk of breast cancer. And once breast cancer is diagnosed, obesity is linked to a higher risk of dying from the disease.

In addition, when fat accumulates around a woman's waistline, there's a stronger relationship to breast cancer as well as heart disease. This so-called "apple shape" — which is characterized by excess abdominal fat — raises insulin levels, which is believed to promote breast cancer cells.[2]

Interestingly, exercising more than three times a week prior to the onset of menopause lowers the risk of breast cancer.[3] It's not necessarily because exercise reduces body fat. The thinking is that exercise can change the length of the menstrual cycle and lower levels of endogenous estrogen and progesterone.

HORMONES FROM OUTSIDE YOUR BODY

Much of our understanding about the role of the body's own hormones in breast cancer came long after pharmaceutical companies started marketing estrogen and progestin drugs. Even so, during the early days of man-made hormones, researchers began to worry that the drugs might be carcinogenic. In her book *The Greatest Experiment Ever Performed on Women,* Barbara Seaman tells of the fears expressed by Charles Dodds, the British chemist who in 1938 developed the first synthetic estrogen — diethylstilbestrol, or DES. Dodds published his formula in the medical journal *Nature* in hopes of thwarting German dominance in the sex hormone market during wartime. Because the formula was published, nobody held the patent, and numerous companies were able to make and market the drug.

According to Seaman, Dodds noticed that male workers in his lab who handled DES were growing breasts, causing him to wonder if the drug might cause breast cancer in men. In 1940, the *Journal of the National Cancer Institute* reported that DES produced breast cancers in male and female mice. Johns Hopkins researchers also published warnings that rats injected with DES and other estrogens developed mammary cancer.[4]

DES is a particularly potent hormone that

is no longer prescribed. Nonetheless, it has a tragic history. The drug was used for some time to prevent miscarriages in pregnant women. Not only did the daughters and sons of those women have a higher risk of certain rare cancers, but the women themselves were at higher risk for breast cancer.

Progestin and the Pill

Despite these warnings, most of the early concerns about hormones and cancer focused on uterine cancer. The risk of uterine cancer in women taking estrogen is so obvious and pronounced it's no wonder it eclipsed fears about breast cancer. In 1975, the *New England Journal of Medicine* reported that the risk of uterine cancer is as much as 14 times higher in estrogen users than in non-estrogen users.

But concerns about breast cancer finally did start to surface. A year after reporting on the risk of uterine cancer, the *New England Journal of Medicine* published a study showing that women who had started estrogen therapy 15 years earlier were twice as likely to develop breast cancer as women who never used estrogen. Again, though, the breast cancer fears didn't really take hold, in part because so much evidence was emerging to show that estrogen was good for a woman's bone health and an effective treatment for osteoporosis. Once reports that menopause hormones protected women against heart disease came to the fore, there was a growing consensus that any small increase in the risk of breast cancer was probably worth the gamble, given the number of lives that hormones could save by reducing heart attacks and hip fractures among aging women.

The worries about uterine cancer were calmed after doctors found that adding progestin to the hormone mix solved the problem. Progestin given in cycles allowed for a regular sloughing off of the uterine lining. Progestin given continuously prevented the building of the uterine lining in the first place. Both methods lower risk of uterine cancer in hormone users.

By adding progestin to the hormone regimen, doctors had protected a woman's uterus but had unknowingly increased her risk of breast cancer. The first sign of this surfaced in 1989, when Swedish researchers reported on a study of more than 23,000 women in which breast cancer was twice as likely to occur in those who used estrogen and progestin than in those who took estrogen alone. Five years later, the *Lancet* published a study by Dutch researchers who were looking at the risk of breast cancer among users of birth control pills. Their study compared 918 women who had been diagnosed with breast cancer between ages 20 and 54 with similar women who were cancer-free. The data suggested that women who used oral contraceptives for more than 12 years were 30 percent more likely to be diagnosed with breast cancer than women who never used the Pill. For women under age 36, the risk among those who used the Pill for 4 years or more was double that of nonusers. Older women between ages 46 and 54 who had used the Pill in the previous 3 years also had nearly double the risk of nonusers.[5]

It's important to note that the birth control pills studied for the *Lancet* report were a far higher dose than the pills prescribed currently, so it's likely that today's oral contraceptives are much safer. Also, menopause drugs contain far lower doses of hormones than birth control pills do. But the research did support the idea that the age at which a woman begins taking hormones and how long she takes them might well be factors in her risk of developing breast cancer.

A Matter of Time

By 1995, the Nurses' Health Study was providing more valuable data on the link between hormone use and breast cancer. The data were important because they came from the same study that had fueled much of the support for menopause hormones with reports that the drugs dramatically lowered a woman's risk of heart disease. This research had begun to show that a woman's risk of breast cancer was strongly associated with how long she used menopause hormones, and that adding progestin likely increased the risk.

The women in the Nurses' Health Study who used estrogen had about a 32 percent higher risk of breast cancer than women who didn't. The women who took estrogen plus progestin saw their risk jump by 41 percent compared with postmenopausal women who never used hormones. Most important, the data showed that women who took hormones for 5 years or more had a 46 percent higher risk of breast cancer. The increase in risk associated with long-term hormone therapy was greatest for older women. Those between the ages of 60 and 64 who used menopause hormones for 5 years or more were 71 percent more likely to develop breast cancer than women their age who didn't use hormones.

Other research strongly supported these conclusions. In October 1997, the *Lancet* reported on research from a collaborative group that had analyzed data collected from more than 150,000 women in 21 countries who were part of 51 different studies. When the data were combined, the researchers concluded that using menopause hormones for 5 years increased breast cancer risk by 35 percent, while using the drugs for more than 5 years boosted risk by 53 percent compared with nonusers. It is important to note that 5 years after women stopped hormones, the higher risk completely disappeared.

While all these percentages sound frightening, they don't actually translate to that big of a risk. As mentioned earlier, a woman's risk of breast cancer is relatively low when she's in her late forties and early fifties. Risk starts to climb as she gets older, peaking in her seventies. So even though hormone use appears to raise breast cancer risk, the Nurses' Health Study in particular showed that the highest risk occurs in the oldest women who are at higher risk to start with.

The best guidance on using menopause hormones has come from the Women's Health Initiative (WHI). While all the previous studies have strongly suggested a link between menopause hormones and breast cancer, with risk increasing the longer a woman uses the drugs, the WHI was the first clinical trial to give us a clear blueprint on the safest way to use these drugs.

The estrogen/progestin segment of the WHI was halted primarily for two reasons: The women who were taking the hormones had higher rates of both heart attacks and breast cancer. From the outset, the investigators who designed the study fully expected the hormone users to have slightly higher breast cancer rates. We already knew fairly convincingly from the Nurses' Health Study and other research that breast cancer was a concern with menopause hormones. The thinking going into the study was that the slightly higher risk of breast cancer would be outweighed by the expected protective effects of hormones in terms of lowering risk of heart attack and hip fracture, among other potential benefits. Sure, some women would be harmed by breast cancer, but far more women were expected to be saved from heart attacks and other health problems. As we discussed in Chapter 4, the way the study was designed, with so many older women starting hormones long past menopause, hormone use resulted in an unexpected surge in heart problems among those older women.

We can only speculate what would have happened had this study tracked younger women starting hormones at the time of menopause. But now we know that older women starting hormones late in life — as they did in the WHI — are at far greater risk for heart attack. As a result, the balance of the safety scale was quickly tipped. The combination of expected breast cancer cases plus increased heart attack risk forced investigators to stop this study early.

Interpreting the Breast Cancer Data

There are a few important flaws to be aware of when trying to make sense of the WHI data. Many of the women had a prior history of hormone use; most did not experience severe hot flashes; and a large percentage of them stopped taking their pills in the midst of the study. All of these factors make it tough to draw definitive conclusions about hormone therapy and breast cancer.

Because the WHI involved mostly older women, many of these women had taken hormones in the past. Some had been on hormone therapy to cope with menopause symptoms, but they stopped treatment several years before joining the WHI study. A small number reported more-recent hormone use, having taken hormones up until the WHI study, then stopping them to join the research. And some women had never taken menopause hormones and did so only because they joined the study.

Most of the women in the larger WHI had never taken hormones; however, 26 percent of those in both hormone studies had. This included about 14 percent who either were current hormone users or had taken hormones in the past for more than 10 years. The problem with this is that the women in the study don't really reflect the type of woman interested in menopause hormones today. The average woman who seeks hormones to treat menopause symptoms is in her late 40s or early 50s, suffers from hot flashes, and has never used menopause hormones. The average woman in the WHI was 63, nearly one-quarter of the women had used menopause hormones in the past, and most of the women weren't suffering from hot flashes when they went on hormones for the study.

Why is this important? Because we already

know that cumulative exposure to menopause hormones increases risk, so many of
the women in the WHI weren't starting at
the same place as the typical hormone user.
Their breasts already had hormone experience, and that may have influenced the results.

There may also be a link between severity
of hot flashes and risk of breast cancer.
Severe hot flashes generally indicate low
estrogen levels, which in turn might signal a
low overall breast cancer risk. We already
know that WHI investigators discouraged
women who had severe hot flashes from
joining the study. So it's possible that the
average woman recruited to the WHI — a
women who did not have severe hot flashes
— was at higher risk for breast cancer to
begin with.

Finally, there was an unusually high
dropout rate in this study. About 40 percent
of the women in both the hormone and the
placebo groups stopped taking their pills.
About 11 percent of the women in the
placebo group who quit the study pills
started taking hormones prescribed by their
doctors. From a statistical standpoint, the
high dropout rate makes it challenging to
interpret the data. It could mean the breast

cancer risk is actually higher than was reported.

What We Can Learn from the WHI

The point is, no study is foolproof, and there are always limits to how reliable any clinical trial data really are. But the WHI has provided the best data we have so far, and with a few exceptions, the data are pretty consistent with the studies that came before it. As a result, despite some of the limitations, we can still learn a lot about menopause hormones and breast cancer risk.

Overall, women in the WHI who took estrogen and progestin had a 24 percent higher risk of breast cancer during the study period. This means that in a group of 20,000 women, if half take combination menopause hormones and half do not, there would be eight additional cases of breast cancer among the hormone users compared with the non-hormone users.[6]

But these data may slightly overstate the risk of hormone use for many women. For a woman deciding whether to use hormones for the first time, the most similar women in the WHI are those who never used menopause hormones before the study. Although these women are much older than the typical woman considering hormone drugs, the fact that their breasts had never before been exposed to menopause hormones makes them similar to the type of woman trying to make her own hormone decision today.

Women in the WHI who had never used menopause hormones but started taking them for the study had a 9 percent higher risk of being diagnosed with breast cancer than women who never used hormones before or during the study. That's far less than the 24 percent overall increase among all women in the study. Other data support the notion that prior hormone use contributed to the risk levels of the women participating in the WHI. Women who had taken hormones for less than 5 years in the past and started using them again had a 70 percent higher risk of breast cancer than women who had never taken hormones. Women with a history of using hormones for more than 5 years, who then resumed treatment for the WHI, doubled their risk of breast cancer compared with similar women in the placebo group.

HORMONES AND MAMMOGRAMS

The WHI demonstrated convincingly that women who take menopause hormones are far more likely to have an unusual mammogram. The reason for this is that menopause hormones increase the density of breast tissue. On a mammogram, it's tough to distinguish dense healthy breast tissue from a tumor, which is also composed of dense tissue. The well-known breast cancer expert Susan Love, MD, likens reading a mammogram of dense breast tissue to "finding a polar bear in a snowstorm."

The problem with breast density and mammograms may explain why the women in the WHI who took both estrogen and progestin seemed to have a lower risk of breast cancer in the first few years of the study. In the first year, the women taking Prempro had a 52 percent lower risk than women who were not taking hormones. In the second year, the hormone users had a 35 percent lower risk. By the third year, the risk among hormone users and nonusers was about equal, with hormone users just 4 percent less likely to develop breast cancer.

In the fourth year, things changed. By then, hormone users had a 45 percent higher risk of breast cancer. The figure jumped to 61 percent by the fifth year. Interestingly, risk started to decline in the sixth year, but it still was 24 percent higher for hormone users than for non-hormone users.[7]

This doesn't necessarily mean that the women who were taking Prempro were at lower risk for breast cancer in the early years of treatment. It's far more likely that their mammograms were harder to read, and as a result, doctors were missing cancers in those years. In the first year of the study, 9 percent of hormone users had abnormal mammograms, while 5 percent of placebo users had abnormal readings.

The reason this is important is that cancer is more easily treated if it's found early. Given that breast cancer generally takes years to develop, it's likely that the women in the WHI were well on their way to developing breast cancer before they joined the study. It's also possible that hormone use then changed the density of their breasts, masking changes that would have alerted doctors to breast cancer sooner.

MORE-SERIOUS CANCERS?

Some early studies have suggested that women who get breast cancer while taking menopause hormones are more likely to get a low-grade cancer that is easier to treat. But these studies may simply be reflecting the fact that women who take hormones are more likely to get regular checkups and mammograms, so their cancers are found earlier compared with women who aren't seeking regular medical care.

Other studies have shown that women on menopause hormones are at higher risk for lobular cancers. Most breast cancers start in the milk duct, but lobular cancer starts in a part of the breast called a lobule. In and of itself, it isn't any more risky than ductal breast cancer. The problem with lobular cancer is that it doesn't form lumps and so is difficult to spot on a mammogram. As a result, it's usually found later than ductal cancer.

This is one big concern with menopause hormones: They not only appear to slightly increase the risk of breast cancer, they also change breast tissue in a way that makes cancers hard to spot. And they are linked with a type of cancer that is also hard to spot. There are potential solutions to these problems, but it's important that women be aware of these complications when deciding whether to use hormones.

ESTROGEN ON ITS OWN

Most scientific research suggests that women who use only estrogen to relieve menopause symptoms have a higher risk of breast cancer than nonusers. Adding progestin to the hormone regimen boosts risk even higher.

But the WHI has challenged — and confused — much of the thinking about estrogen and breast cancer.

Although the arm of the WHI looking at estrogen and progestin was stopped early because of a higher risk of breast cancer and heart troubles among the hormone users, those problems didn't occur in the second arm of the trial — the one that involved women who took estrogen alone because they had undergone hysterectomies. Eventually, the estrogen-only part of the study was stopped early as well, but it was a controversial decision that even the WHI's own data safety monitoring board didn't agree with. Officials from the National Heart, Lung, and Blood Institute made the decision, citing a slightly increased risk of stroke and blood clots among estrogen users. (These risks will be discussed in future chapters.)

The problem with this decision is that the estrogen-only arm of the WHI was producing some exciting data. Not only had the women taking estrogen avoided the heart attack risk that showed up in the combination hormone trial, but their breast cancer risk was a whopping 20 percent lower than that of women who weren't taking hormones.[8] Because the trial was stopped early, we don't have enough data to draw definitive conclusions, so we don't fully understand what this trend means.

Some additional analyses of the available data raise the possibility that estrogen may indeed offer protection. Because 54 percent of the women in the WHI had stopped taking their pills by the end of the study, investigators decided to also analyze data collected from just those women who consistently took their medications. This group showed a 33 percent lower risk of breast cancer — a trend that is considered statistically valid. When the investigators looked at specific cancers, estrogen appeared to reduce the risk of ductal carcinoma — the most common type of breast cancer — by 29 percent.[9]

So why did earlier studies show conflicting results?

Most of the data suggesting estrogen users have a higher risk of breast cancer come from observational studies conducted 20 to 25 years ago. Mammography screening at that time wasn't as common as it is today. And in an observational study, you don't tell women to get a mammogram. You just watch large groups of people and pay attention to the different patterns that emerge.

Observational studies have shown that estrogen users have a higher risk of breast cancer. But we know that women who take estrogen are more likely to get regular medical care, including screening mammograms. So could it be that the higher breast cancer risk reported among estrogen users all these years simply reflects the fact that estrogen users are more likely to get mammograms? You are more likely to find cancer in women if you are looking for it, so it makes sense that you are more likely to find breast cancer in estrogen users who get mammograms than in non-estrogen users who don't get mammograms. Obviously, doctors will eventually detect breast cancer in women who don't get mammograms, but it's not clear if those delayed diagnoses will be discovered in time to influence the earlier study data.

More-recent observational studies among women who get regular mammograms show that those who use estrogen alone may have a lower risk of breast cancer. In 2004, for example, the *Journal of Clinical Oncology* published a report from researchers in San Francisco and Seattle. In this study of nearly 375,000 postmenopausal women who frequented community-based mammography practices, the researchers found that the women who took estrogen for more than 5 years had an 8 percent lower risk of breast cancer than nonusers. Because false-negative rates were the same among both groups, researchers say it's unlikely that delays in diagnosis (like those seen in the estrogen/progestin segment of the WHI) are a problem with this group of women. Moreover, the women in the study who took estrogen and progestin for more than 5 years had a 49 percent higher risk of breast cancer than nonusers,[10] while the women who used estrogen and progestin for less than 5 years were not at increased risk — trends that are markedly similar to those found in the WHI.

Still, several quirks in the WHI study population make it hard to draw definitive conclusions about whether taking estrogen really lowers a woman's risk of breast cancer. For instance, nearly half of the women in the estrogen-only study were obese, so it's possible that the results are less applicable to women who are thin. Because fat is a source of estrogen, it may be that women who are overweight have so much natural estrogen from fat that adding more from pills doesn't make much difference.

152

Some researchers have suggested that the differences between the two study groups in the WHI strongly support the notion that progestin is the real culprit behind the increased breast cancer risk from hormone use. Some believe that the type of progestin studied — medroxyprogesteron acetate, or MPA — is too potent and that progesterone pills more similar to a woman's natural progesterone would lessen the negative effects on breast cancer. Others think the problem is that the WHI used continuous progestin — meaning women took progestin every day along with estrogen — rather than a cyclic progestin that women take only a few days a month, thus lowering their overall exposure to progestin. These are important questions to which we don't have definitive answers. And we don't know if it's really the individual progestin that is the problem, or some interaction between progestin and estrogen that is creating the higher breast cancer risk.

An important British study, called the Million Women Study, looked at women using a number of different types of progestin regimens. It didn't find any differences in breast cancer risk.[11] Women certainly have the option of choosing different hormone regimens than those studied in the WHI. I will explore questions about progestin, as well as different estrogen products, in Chapters 11 and 12. That said, most experts believe that until we know more, women should assume all progestins carry the same risks.

THE ROLE OF ALCOHOL

Alcohol consumption is an important risk factor for breast cancer, particularly for postmenopausal women. It's confusing because women have heard a lot about how moderate alcohol consumption helps their hearts. It does. But it also hurts their breasts.

The American Cancer Society Prevention Study, which followed American women for 14 years, reported that consuming less than one drink a day on average increased a post-menopausal woman's chances of dying from breast cancer by 30 percent compared with women who did not consume any alcohol.[12] More research is needed to determine whether premenopausal women have a higher risk of breast cancer as a result of alcohol use, but some studies suggest this is the case.[13]

It's not clear how much alcohol it takes to increase a woman's chances of getting breast cancer. The average woman has a lifetime risk of breast cancer of about one in eight, or 12.5 percent. One study showed that for the average woman who has one drink a day, the chances of being diagnosed with breast cancer during her lifetime would increase to about one in seven, or about 14.25 percent.[14]

Another study compared alcohol consumption between women in the United States and Italy. In the United States, alcohol is linked to about 1 in 50 cases of breast cancer each year. In Italy, where women consume more alcohol, about 1 in 6 breast cancers is thought to be alcohol related.[15]

Alcohol adds considerably to a woman's breast cancer risk if she also takes menopause hormones. A study published in the *Annals of Internal Medicine* in 2002 looked at data from 44,000 women in the Nurses' Health Study, which showed that alcohol by itself raised risk. Women who consumed one to two drinks a day but didn't use menopause hormones were 28 percent more likely to develop breast cancer than similar women who consumed no alcohol. But women who use both alcohol and hormones faced even greater risk. Those who took menopause hormones for 5 years or more and also consumed one to two alcoholic beverages a day were nearly twice as likely to develop breast cancer as those who didn't drink or take hormones. According to the study, a hypothetical postmenopausal woman whose lifetime risk of breast cancer is 4 percent could increase her risk to 8 percent with 5 years of hormone use and alcohol consumption exceeding one drink a day.[16]

How to Determine Your Personal Risk

The average woman has a one in eight chance of developing breast cancer in her lifetime. But that's an average. Many women have a far lower risk.

Women who have a family history of breast cancer or who are known to carry a specific gene associated with breast cancer obviously have a higher-than-normal risk. Women who have already been diagnosed with breast cancer are at risk for recurrence. These factors — as well as the other risks and benefits associated with menopause hormones — must be taken into account as a woman is trying to decide whether to use hormones.

The final chapter of this book will attempt to help you weigh all the risks and benefits of hormones. But many women are most concerned about breast cancer. For this reason, it may be useful to try to gauge your personal risk of breast cancer. Once you've established your baseline risk, you can get a better sense of what some of the risks associated with hormone use will mean for you.

It's hard to know how much hormone therapy could add to your personal risk of breast cancer. The WHI showed that women who never used hormones had only a 9 percent increase in risk over a 5-year period, but observational studies have suggested about a 30 percent increase in risk. A 30 percent increase due to hormone use sounds scary until you do the math. For instance, a relatively healthy 50-year-old woman may find that her chances of being diagnosed with breast cancer in the next 5 years are less than 2 percent. Even factoring in a 30 percent increase in risk from hormone use, her overall risk for being diagnosed with breast cancer during the next 5 years would still be less than 3 percent. Depending on her other health concerns, that slight increase in overall risk may be an easy trade-off. At the same time, a woman who discovers that her short-term risk is higher than expected may decide the benefits of menopause hormones aren't worth the other risks she faces.

As we have discussed, individual risk of breast cancer is influenced by many factors we can never control or can no longer change — such as a woman's age at her first period, her age at the birth of her first child, whether she breastfed, and her age at menopause. The age at which a woman begins taking birth control pills and how long she takes them will alter her risk, as will prior menopause hormone use. The density of a woman's breasts and past history of benign breast disease also play a role. There are some risk factors we can change, however, such as how often we exercise, whether or not we consume alcohol — and whether or not we use menopause hormones.

Two Web sites provide useful calculators that will help you assess and understand your personal risk of breast cancer. The first Web site, www.cancer.gov/bcrisktool/, allows you to input some basic information about your health, from which it will calculate your baseline risk of breast cancer before using menopause hormones. Once you have a number, you can do your own math to figure out if the risks and benefits of these drugs are worth it to you. The second Web site, www.yourdiseaserisk.com, won't give you a number, but it will show you a useful bar graph and where you fall on the risk spectrum, from low to high. What's great about this Web site, created by researchers from the Harvard Center for Cancer Prevention, is that it factors in recent data about the risks of menopause hormones. You can look at your risk before using hormones, then go back and add menopause hormones into your profile to see how your risk changes.

YOUR HORMONE DECISION

In deciding whether to use menopause hormones, you need to weigh all the risks, not just breast cancer. Your overall menopause symptoms, your risk for osteoporosis, and other health concerns that are influenced by hormones should be part of your decision. In terms of hormone use and breast cancer risk specifically, recent studies have given us some important guidance.

Estrogen and progestin. We know that women who use estrogen and progestin have a slightly higher risk of breast cancer. If you are a woman experiencing natural menopause and considering taking estrogen and progestin, the best way to minimize your breast cancer risk is to limit use of these drugs to less than 5 years. Ideally, you would take them for 3 years or less, as

159

reflected by the WHI data.

Taking menopause hormones likely will result in an increase in breast density that may make a standard mammogram less reliable. Studies show that women with dense breasts benefit from having mammograms annually rather than every 2 years. In addition, if you choose to take menopause hormones, you might consider talking to your doctor about a breast sonogram, which does a better job of finding trouble spots in dense breasts, as well as the lobular cancers that are more likely to occur in hormone users.

Estrogen alone. Women who have undergone hysterectomies and take only estrogen may have a slightly lower risk of breast cancer or at least no increase in risk. Though not conclusive, the WHI data — coupled with recent observational study data — should be reassuring to women considering this treatment. The WHI showed that women who had undergone hysterectomies could safely take estrogen for up to 7 years without raising their risk of breast cancer.

A new analysis of data from the Nurses' Health Study has given us even more information about how long women can safely take estrogen. Among more than 28,000 nurses, there was no statistically significant increase in breast cancer risk through 20 years of estrogen use. After 20 years, risk jumped by 42 percent. Among cancers that have both estrogen and progesterone receptors — which accounted for 44 percent of the cancer cases — breast cancer risk rose sooner, at the 15-year mark.

Fifteen to 20 years is far longer than most women would use estrogen. Most experts still recommend short-term estrogen therapy. But for women who had their ovaries removed at a young age, who've undergone cancer treatment or early menopause, or who continue to have difficult menopause symptoms after five years, the data from the Nurses' Health Study should be reassuring.[17]

Breast cancer isn't the only health issue to think about when making decisions about hormone use. Let's move on to some other body parts.

6
HORMONES AND
YOUR BONES

Here's a depressing statistic: When it comes to building bone, it's all downhill after 30. That's the age at which women reach their peak bone mass — meaning it's the last year in a woman's life that her body is building more bone than it's losing. So by the time you start coping with the symptoms of menopause, your bones have already undergone 2 decades of steady decline. For most women, this is just normal aging and nothing to worry about. But for a small minority of women, bone health is a serious health issue. Menopause hormones are one option for protecting fragile bones as we age.

Bones are living tissue, just like the heart, lungs, and other organs. The body builds bone at a frenzied pace in our infancy. This process slows down for a while in childhood, then picks up again in adolescence. That's why a healthful calcium-rich diet, weight-bearing exercise, and not smoking are so important for kids: It's the time in life when lifestyle choices can have the biggest impact on bone health. The body is pretty much done with bone building by age 18, though it continues to fine-tune and make minor additions for another decade. Hormones — estrogen in women and testosterone in men — help drive this building boom in our youth.

After 3 decades of mostly building, the body shifts into "remodeling" mode. Remodeling happens around the clock; it's the continuous breakdown and reformation of bone. And it's controlled by hormones.

The process of breaking down bone is called resorption. It's performed by osteoclasts, large cells that live in the center of the bone. The osteoclasts remove microscopic bits of bone. Then bone-forming cells called osteoblasts replace the lost bone with new bone. The problem is that the osteoclasts are better at removing bone than the osteoblasts are at building it. This gap is the reason that we all slowly lose bone as we age.

A woman's bone story gets worse as she reaches menopause, whether naturally or due to surgery or radiation treatments. Either way, the body loses its once-plentiful estrogen supply from the ovaries. Remember that the bone-building and remodeling process is controlled by hormones, including estrogen. Once estrogen is in short supply, the rate of bone loss speeds up for about 5 to 8 years. Estrogen is essentially the construction site foreman, telling the osteoblast workers to get moving and start building bone. Without the hormone there to shout orders, the osteoblasts get lazy. But the osteoclasts keep working hard, removing bits of bone. As a result, more bone is lost than formed.

Is Losing Bone a Serious Health Worry?

Before you factor the bone benefits of estrogen into your hormone decision, you have to determine whether osteoporosis and fracture risk are serious health concerns for you. Losing more bone than your body makes sounds like a dire predicament that will leave you broken by the time you are 60. But for the majority of women, this loss of bone density over time and particularly at menopause doesn't translate into any real health problem. Most of us build up a nice little cushion of bone density in our youth, so even though it starts to diminish in our thirties, we have plenty to work with. Once bone loss speeds up in menopause, some women are at higher risk for problems, but the vast majority of women will be fine well into their seventies and eighties.

That doesn't mean that bone health isn't something to pay attention to. Fractures of the hip, wrist, and spine are all concerns for elderly women. Broken bones don't heal as quickly when we're older. Spine fractures can leave you hunched over; a broken hip can result in loss of mobility, confinement to a nursing home, or even death. So bone health is obviously important. But a lot of people question whether low bone density related to estrogen loss and normal aging is the main reason bones are vulnerable to breaking when we get older. Some medical experts speculate that the risks of low bone density may have been hyped by drug companies who want to sell their treatments, and by doctors and medical technology companies who have invested heavily in bone-density scanning equipment. If women aren't worried about bone health, they won't get bone-density tests.

Part of the problem is that we have a tendency to compare women past 50 with women in their twenties and thirties. Few 50-year-old women look the same as they did at 20, nor do they necessarily want to. But a diagnosis of low bone-density typically is based on how a woman's bones look in a bone-density scan compared with the bones of a 20- or 30-year-old. Women who go for bone-density screenings may hear about "T-scores" or "standard deviations" or "minus 1" measurements. The bottom line is that a woman is considered to have low bone density if her bones are more than one standard deviation below a younger woman's. This doesn't mean she's unhealthy. It just means her bones have gone through the same normal aging process as everyone else's.

Even so, the osteoporosis industry has come up with a scary-sounding name for normal aging bones: *osteopenia.* If your doctor tells you that you have osteopenia, don't be alarmed. It means that you don't have unusually high bone density for your age, and you don't have unusually brittle bones. Most of the time, it just means you're normal.

WHAT IS OSTEOPOROSIS?

The definition of osteoporosis has evolved over the years, and the changes have fueled a growing skepticism about how much of a health worry osteoporosis really is for most women. In the past, a woman wasn't considered to have osteoporosis unless she had already suffered a fracture due to weak bones. Today, the definition is broader. Osteoporosis is a disease characterized by low bone mass that makes a woman more susceptible to fractures.

A woman who gets a bone-density scan will learn her T-score, a number that's meant to indicate her level of bone health. For a postmenopausal woman, a score of up to minus 1.0 is normal. A score between minus 1.0 and minus 2.5 is classified as osteopenia or low bone density. Anything below a minus 2.5 is considered osteoporosis.

According to the National Osteoporosis Foundation, 20 percent of white and Asian women age 50 and older are believed to have osteoporosis. So are 10 percent of Hispanic women and 5 percent of African American women. Think about these numbers for a moment. They mean that 80 to 95 percent of women *don't* have osteoporosis.

Bone Density and Osteoporosis Risk

The osteoporosis industry will tell you that women with low bone density are also at risk. It is true that the lower your bone density, the higher your risk of fracture. But risk is all relative. Just because your risk is higher than that of a 30-year-old woman doesn't mean you're likely to suffer a hip fracture. It just means that the risk of various health problems changes as we get older. We won't start dropping like flies as soon as we reach 50.

In fact, often a woman's age matters more than her bone density. In 2002, a World Health Organization study looked at 10-year risk of hip fracture among women around the world.[1] Risk varied widely depending on country, diet, activity level, health status, and numerous other factors. The typical 50-year-old American woman has less than a 1 percent chance of experiencing a hip fracture over the next 10 years. When she reaches 60, her risk jumps to 1.8 percent. At 70, her risk is 5 percent. If she lives past 80, her risk of a hip fracture in the next decade rises to 14.2 percent.

All this attention to estrogen loss, low bone density, and osteoporosis risk may be sending the wrong health message. Women who have low bone density may be overly fearful about fracture risk, while women who have good bone density aren't paying enough attention to their bone health.

An important study published in the *New England Journal of Medicine* in 1995 looked at 9,516 white women age 65 or older who had never had a hip fracture. (The incidence of hip facture is twice as high among white women as among African American women.) The study followed these women for more than 4 years, checking in with them every 4 months to gauge their fracture risk. The researchers found that while low bone density is a risk factor for breaking bones, it's not the only risk factor. Some women with high bone density still suffer broken bones.[2]

Questions to Ask about Your Bones

What's so important about this study is that it gives us practical information for gauging our own bone health even if we haven't had a bone scan. While the research confirmed that bone density is important, it clearly shows that bone density is not the only issue to think about. Further, it identifies numerous factors that put a woman at risk for suffering fractures as she gets older.

What's your family history? Some of the most important information we get about our bone health comes from our mothers. If your mother had a hip fracture, your risk is double that of a woman without the family history. Women in the *New England Journal* study whose mothers suffered hip fractures before age 80 were nearly three times as likely to suffer a hip fracture themselves. For women in this group, bone density isn't the biggest indicator of risk. If your mother suffered a hip fracture, your risk of hip fracture is the same, regardless of whether you have high or low bone density.

Thin or fat? Carrying a few extra pounds seems to protect a woman from hip fracture, while being thin increases her risk. Bone protection isn't a big enough benefit to justify weight gain. But knowing your weight-gain patterns can help you gauge your bone health. The more weight a woman had gained since age 25, the lower her risk of hip fracture. Women who weigh less than they did at 25 had twice the risk of hip fracture.

How far do you fall? Women who were tall at age 25 also had a greater risk of hip fracture. Height may be a risk factor because tall women fall farther and harder. Or there could be something with the hip architecture of a tall woman that puts her at higher risk of fracture when she does fall.

Do you drink coffee, tea, and cola? The more caffeine a woman drinks, the more likely she is to suffer a hip fracture. Caffeine leeches calcium from your bones.

Still standing? Women who spent no more than 4 hours a day on their feet had twice the risk of hip fracture compared with women who spent more time standing and walking.

Still moving? Women who regularly walked for exercise had a 30 percent lower risk of hip fracture than women who did not walk regularly. Risk goes down the farther you walk, dropping nearly 1 percent for every five blocks. Overall, being in poor physical condition raises risk. Another important finding that emerged from the *New England Journal* study: Women who couldn't rise from a chair without using their arms were at a two-fold higher risk for hip fracture.

Are other things breaking? Fracturing any bone after age 50 signals a higher risk of hip fracture after menopause, regardless of bone density.

What's your bone density? Low bone density increased hip fracture risk by 60 percent. But many women with low bone density didn't suffer fractures. Women in the study with low bone density and no more than one other risk factor had just a 2.6 percent risk of hip fracture in a given year. By comparison, women with high bone density had a 9 percent annual risk of hip fracture if they had at least five other risk factors.

In fact, it's having a combination of risk

factors that may be most important in determining a woman's risk of hip fracture. For example, among women with two or fewer risk factors, the rate of hip fracture was only 1.1 per 1,000 women each year. Women with five or more risk factors but not low bone density had 19 fractures per 1,000 women. The group with five or more risk factors *and* low bone density were at highest risk, with 27 hip fractures per 1,000 women.[3]

This research shows that while low bone density is a factor in our bone health as we age, it alone doesn't doom us to certain fractures. Nor does high bone density guarantee protection from the perils of broken bones. In the *New England Journal* study, only 6 percent of women were at the highest risk for hip fracture. These women had a number of risk factors in addition to low bone density, and they accounted for 62 percent of all the fractures in the study.

What does this tell us? Most of us don't need to worry too much about hip fracture. The medical community's focus should be on women who have both low bone density and several of the other known risk factors for hip fracture.

The story of menopause hormones and how they help protect bones starts in 1941, when Harvard researcher Fuller Albright, MD, published a report in the *Journal of the American Medical Association* suggesting that estrogen might stimulate bone formation. He noted that women whose ovaries are surgically removed in their twenties or thirties quickly lose bone mass, with some developing osteoporosis before age 40. He suggested that estrogen drugs to replace a woman's diminished natural estrogen might be a solution for women who lost ovarian function at a young age.[4] While the medical community has been quick to embrace other purported benefits of hormone drugs, it was uncharacteristically cautious about this one.

Things changed in 1982 when a San Francisco radiologist published research on 27 premenopausal women who experienced surgical menopause as a result of having their ovaries removed. The women were given different doses of Premarin or a placebo. The women who took the highest dose, 0.625 milligram of Premarin (which is the same amount used by the women in the Women's Health Initiative), retained much of their bone mass. The women on lower doses of estrogen or the placebo lost bone. Even though the study involved women who had undergone surgical menopause, the finding led directly to a widespread publicity effort by makers of hormone drugs to raise awareness about osteoporosis and bone loss associated with menopause.[5]

Until recently, the effect of menopause hormones on bone health wasn't known. The Women's Health Initiative (WHI) marked the first time anyone had demonstrated not only that estrogen drugs improve bone density but also that the improved bone mass translates into a lower risk of broken bones. When the study results were announced in July 2002, the benefits of menopause hormones to bone health were virtually ignored as national health officials, doctors, and women themselves paid far more attention to the various risks of hormone therapy. But people who had been following bone health research for decades were shocked at just how much impact menopause hormones have on frail bones.

Women in the WHI who took estrogen and progestin had a 33 percent lower risk of hip fracture.[6] Women in the estrogen-only segment of the trial showed a 35 percent reduction in risk if they took the hormone.[7] The benefits were even greater in certain groups.

Other issues that affected fracture risk included calcium intake and body size. Women who used estrogen and progestin showed a 60 percent reduction in risk if they also took 1,200 milligrams of calcium a day. Thin women — those with a body mass index of less than 25 — had a 50 percent reduction in risk with hormone therapy. Women with a body mass index between 25 and 30 had a 23 percent reduction in risk, and women with a body mass index above 30 didn't show any benefit.

One of the most surprising findings to come out of the WHI recently was that the risk-benefit equation is different for women at high risk for bone fracture compared with everyone else. WHI investigators concluded that among older women, the risk of heart problems, breast cancer, stroke, and blood clots outweighed any benefits, particularly the reduction in risk of hip fracture. However, a study published in the *Journal of the American Medical Association* in 2003 calculated whether women at high risk for fracture might have more to gain from hormone use. The researchers used a global index, weighing all the risks and benefits of hormone therapy. For women at low or moderate risk for hip fracture, the bone health benefits weren't enough to negate the other risks, so their overall risk of health problems was still 20 percent higher than for women who didn't use hormones. But the story was different for women at high risk for fracture. Comparing all the risks and benefits for these women, hormone use increased their overall risk of health problems by just 3 percent.[8] This means that using hormones so dramatically lowered the risk of serious fractures that the bone benefit virtually negated all the other risks associated with hormone therapy in older women.

BUT DOES IT LAST?

So now we know that menopause hormones boost bone health. But most experts recommend against long-term use of these drugs because of other health concerns that may be associated with them. The question is whether the benefits to bone density from using hormones stick around once a woman stops taking the drugs. Unfortunately, the answer seems to be no.

In 2003, researchers from the University of California, San Diego, reported on 170,852 postmenopausal women ages 50 to 104 who were not known to have osteoporosis. They compared current hormone use, past hormone use, and fracture risk to gauge whether hormone therapy has a lasting impact on bone health. Women who were using hormones at the time of the study had the highest bone density at every age. Current users were 25 percent less likely to suffer a fracture during the yearlong study than non-hormone users. And the longer a woman had used hormones, the higher her bone density — but only as long as she was still taking the drugs. Women who had stopped using menopause hormones more than 5 years earlier had similar bone-density scores to women who had never used hormones.[9] Even among former users who had been on hormone drugs for years, there was no difference in bone health compared with women who had never been on the drugs.

Although hormone use clearly has an immediate impact on bone health, the researchers concluded that using menopause hormones for 5 years or less to treat menopause symptoms is unlikely to preserve bone or significantly reduce fracture risk in later years. This means that if you are taking hormones, your bones are safer than if you aren't taking hormones. But once you stop the drugs, the benefits disappear.

While menopause hormones are proven to reduce fracture risk, the dilemma is that the most benefit occurs among older women and with long-term use. Older women are the ones at highest risk for weak bones, but as we've seen in earlier chapters, older women could face other dangers if they start taking hormones just to protect their bones. We've also seen that in those women at high risk for bone fracture, the bone benefits of hormones almost entirely erase other risks associated with hormone use. But that's relevant to only a small number of women. For most women, improved bone health is not a good reason to start taking hormones.

In the wake of the WHI, however, a new push is on to determine if low doses of estrogen can protect a woman's bones without increasing her risk of other problems. The FDA has approved a new low-dose estrogen patch for use in osteoporosis prevention. The patch, called Menostar, delivers a tiny dose of estrogen — just 14 micrograms a day. That's half the dose of most estrogen-patch drugs and about four times less estrogen than is delivered in conventional hormone treatments.

In a 2-year study, researchers funded by the drug company that makes the patch found that this tiny dose of estrogen still increased bone density by about 3 percent in women's spines and by nearly 1 percent in their hips.[10] We don't know if the improvement in bone density is enough to actually prevent fractures. But we can compare the bone-density benefits of the low-dose patch with the benefits seen in the WHI. We know that women in the WHI who experienced improvement in bone density also experienced a meaningful reduction in their real-life risk of fracture. In the WHI, menopause hormones improved spine bone density by 3.3 percent and hip bone density by 2.1 percent after 1 year of treatment. After 3 years, bone density jumped by 4.5 percent in the spine and by 3.6 percent in the hip.

In terms of spine density, the results of the low-dose patch come pretty close to matching the results of the hormones in the WHI. As for hip density, the patch produced only about half the improvement seen with the higher-dose drugs in the WHI. In addition, there's no evidence right now that women who are coping with hot flashes and other menopause symptoms will find relief with this low-dose patch.

Women concerned about bone health need to be aware that other drugs besides hormones are available to protect bones. Exercise, weight loss, calcium supplements, drugs called bisphosphonates, and so-called designer estrogens are all non-hormone options for boosting bone health. We will explore these in Chapter 13, which will look at drug treatments and alternative therapies for various menopausal health concerns.

Your Hormone Decision

The story of estrogen, bone loss, and menopause hormones is a complicated one. Menopause hormones provide clear benefits to women in terms of improving bone health. The dilemma is that the biggest benefit likely occurs for older women and with long-term use. As we have discussed in previous chapters, older women shouldn't start taking these drugs to prevent other health problems. And there's a lot of uncertainty about the real risks and benefits of using these drugs for 5 years or more. Further, any bone benefits from hormone use are temporary and disappear once a woman stops taking the drugs. As a result, for most women, bone health is not a good reason to take regular menopause hormones.

However, women at high risk for bone fractures have more to gain from menopause hormones than the rest of us. Although studies show that for these women, the bone benefits mostly outweigh other potential risks, it remains a matter of medical debate as to whether fracture prevention justifies long-term hormone use by women with weak bones. Other drugs can boost a woman's bone health, but they carry their own set of side effects, risks, and benefits.

The new, low-dose estrogen patch may be a good option for women worried about osteoporosis. The patch does improve bone density, but as yet, there's no proof that it reduces fracture risk or that it works to treat any other menopause symptoms.

7
HORMONES AND
YOUR VAGINA

Hot flashes get all the attention, but during the menopausal transition, much of the action is happening in and around your vagina.

The most obvious changes involve your period. The cycle may become shorter, longer, or unpredictable. Some months, you may have two periods; other months, you may have no period at all. Eventually, it will be gone long enough (12 months) that your doctor will declare you officially past menopause. But that doesn't mean the experience is over.

Along with noticeable changes in the pattern of your period, you may detect subtle changes in your vaginal health. You may be aroused and interested in sex with your partner, but your vagina doesn't cooperate. There's less vaginal lubrication, and sex just isn't as effortless as it used to be. Without the lubrication, you may develop burning and itching, and sex might become painful.

Not everyone will experience these problems, but they are relatively common during the menopausal transition. A University of Melbourne study found that only about 3 percent of women in their reproductive years complain about vaginal dryness, and just 4 percent notice the problem at the beginning of the menopausal transition. But by the time women are well on their way to menopause, 21 percent complain of vaginal problems. The number jumps to 47 percent after menopause.[1] So even if you don't have problems right now, eventually you may be among the roughly half of women who experience vaginal dryness or discomfort as they age.

Along with changes in your vagina, you may notice changes in your sex life around menopause. These changes may be due in part to vaginal dryness; after all, if sex takes a lot of effort and involves pain, many women and their partners start to lose interest. But the sex life of a menopausal woman isn't defined only by her hormones. To be sure, hormonal fluctuations often play a role in her level of interest and sexual satisfaction. But numerous studies show that sex is far more complicated than that.

Other menopausal symptoms, like hot

flashes and sleep problems, can leave you feeling exhausted and uninterested in sex. Weight gain during menopause can affect your self-esteem and dampen your enthusiasm for a naked romp. The challenges of midlife — teenagers, aging parents, job demands — can all affect sexual interest and satisfaction. So, too, can how long you've been married, how you feel about your partner, your partner's own sexual health, and whether you are having an affair or are in a new relationship.

NATURAL ESTROGEN AND THE AGING OF THE VAGINA

As a woman ages and her hormone levels drop, one of the most obvious differences is a change in her menstrual cycle and bleeding patterns. Up to 90 percent of women experience some change in menstruation during the menopausal transition. The closer you get to menopause, the more likely your menstrual cycles will grow longer before they disappear altogether.[2]

As a woman's ovarian function changes, the level of circulating estradiol — the most common estrogen in the body before menopause — drops dramatically. Since cells with estrogen receptors appear throughout the body, the five- to ten-fold reduction in circulating estradiol has a profound impact throughout the body. Among the possible changes are reduced blood flow to the vaginal area, thinning of the vaginal wall, weakening of the vaginal muscles, and changes in vaginal pH.[3] A woman's reproductive organs and genitals may get smaller, and her skin and mucous membranes will get thinner. Changes also occur in the urinary tract, as bladder size, the thickness of the membrane lining the bladder, and urethra and pelvic muscle tone all are affected.[4] Other potential changes include increased risk of vaginal infections and urinary tract infections, which can lead to an increased risk of arousal disorders and sexual pain disorders. Vaginal spasms, urinary incontinence, and bleeding after sex also can occur.

While all this sounds pretty terrible, don't be alarmed. Many of these changes, while measurable in a research setting, don't always translate into problems for women in real life. In some women, some of the changes, including vaginal dryness, may be transient — bothersome while you're in the throes of the menopausal transition but resolving once your hormones calm down.

Lorraine Dennerstein, a psychiatrist and head of the Melbourne Women's Midlife

Health Project, which has generated much of what we know about women's sexual health during menopause, notes that vaginal dryness isn't always a negative. Your body still produces lubrication; it may just take more effort. The problem often can be solved simply by taking a little more time to reach arousal before having sex. The extra foreplay can actually improve sexual relationships, notes Dr. Dennerstein.

Indeed, some women report that they prefer sex after menopause, even with all the physical changes going on in their bodies. For the first time in years, they discover that intimacy can be stress-free. The kids have moved out of the house, and a woman no longer has to cope with periods or worries about getting pregnant.

ESTROGEN THERAPY AND YOUR VAGINA

To understand why women experience vaginal changes during the menopausal transition, it helps to learn a little bit about what happens when a woman is sexually stimulated. Sexual response is complex and obviously involves more than just a woman's genitals, but sexual stimulation triggers a cascade of changes in a woman's body. Smooth muscles in the genital tissues, including the vagina and clitoris, begin to relax. The relaxation triggers increased blood flow, causing genital tissues to engorge. The vaginal canal increases in length and width, the labia swells, and small glands inside the vagina release lubricant to prepare it for intercourse.[5]

For a woman's genitals to undergo these changes, sustain them for sex, and then return to their natural state, the vaginal tissues need to be strong and pliable. Much of this strength and elasticity is influenced by estrogen. A woman's genital tissues have a high number of estrogen receptors. Estrogen helps these tissues stay plump and maintain their structure. It also plays a role in how these tissues function.

And so, when a woman's natural estrogen starts to wane, tissues in the vaginal area begin to thin and lose their size, shape, and color. There's also less blood flow and lubrication. When estrogen is in short supply, the vagina doesn't ready itself for intercourse, and attempts at sex can be uncomfortable and painful.

Various studies show that estrogen therapy is effective in preserving and restoring vaginal health, relieving vaginal dryness, itching, burning, and pain.[6] The Women's Health Initiative (WHI), which was designed to examine the long-term heart effects of hormone use, didn't directly measure the impact of menopause hormones on vaginal health. But other respected studies show that women who are taking hormones in pills or patches to cope with hot flashes and other menopausal symptoms likely will have improved vaginal health as well. Some women may opt for vaginal creams or tablets or vaginal or intrauterine rings that release hormones directly to the affected area.

Just as with other body parts, the timing of hormone therapy may be important. Whether women use hormones just as their vaginal health is changing or they wait until well after menopause to seek treatment may make a difference in how the vagina responds. Researchers examining vaginal cells from women before and after menopause found that the cells respond differently to estrogen. Treating postmenopausal cells only partially restored their function, while the function of premenopausal cells was fully restored.[7] This basically means that the vagina doesn't bounce back completely if it's been starved of estrogen for a while. The data suggest that the earlier estrogen is used, the better the vaginal cells respond.[8]

While estrogen clearly makes a difference in vaginal health after menopause, it's not the only option for women. Non-hormonal vaginal lubricants and moisturizers have been shown in some studies to be just as effective as hormonal creams.[9] It's also important to note that simply having sex fairly often appears to improve vaginal health. Women who are more sexually active are less likely to experience vaginal atrophy as they age. It's the "use it or lose it" effect. Nobody knows exactly why this is. One study compared postmenopausal women who had sex three or more times a month with women who had sex fewer than 10 times a year. The sexually active women had healthier, younger vaginas than the sexually inactive women.[10]

MENOPAUSE AND YOUR SEX LIFE

Before you worry too much about the toll of declining estrogen levels on your vagina, remember that hormones are only one part of the story. A voluminous body of research shows that declining estrogen is just one factor in your sexual health as you age, and it's not even the most important factor in determining your sexual happiness.

The Melbourne Women's Midlife Health Project found that one of the biggest determinants of sexual function during menopause is a woman's sexual function prior to menopause.[11] If you have an active, satisfying sex life before menopause, chances are you will continue to do so, even with the changes brought on by declining estrogen levels. If you have hang-ups about sex, you're in a bad relationship, or you just weren't that sexually active during your reproductive years, then things will stay pretty much the same — or get worse — during menopause unless you try to resolve the underlying issues that are hampering your sex life.

The second most important factor in your sex life during menopause is your partner. It sounds simple and obvious, but you have to like your partner to be happy with your sex life. Vaginal changes and arousal problems can be a frustrating part of aging, but they won't necessarily have a huge impact on your sexual happiness if you love the one you're with.

However, being in a long-term, stable relationship doesn't guarantee a good sex life during menopause. Researchers studying 2,109 women between ages 40 and 69 found that women in a significant relationship had sex more frequently. But being in a significant relationship also correlated with higher levels of sexual dysfunction.[12]

For any woman in a long-term relationship, it's not entirely surprising that sexual interest can start to wane. Notably, one of the biggest determinants of a good sex life during menopause is whether you have a new partner.[13] That's not to say you can't have a satisfying sex life if you're in a long-term relationship. But women who change partners are more likely to notice changes in their sex lives. Some researchers call this the "in love" effect. Meeting someone new triggers changes in the brain and bursts of dopamine that are partly responsible for all the excitement you feel in a new relationship. A new partner can more than double your sexual responsiveness and boost your libido.[14] Obviously, changing partners isn't a desirable or plausible option for most menopausal women.

The main lesson here is that if you are unhappy with your sex life, you shouldn't immediately blame menopause. Your personal sex history is the biggest factor in your sex life after menopause. The quality of your relationship matters, too. "If there are negative feelings toward the partner — anger or resentment going back perhaps many years over many different things — that is going to have a far more powerful effect at any stage of the woman's life than the hormonal changes of menopause," says Dr. Denner-stein.[15]

HORMONES AND YOUR SEX LIFE

So whether or not your sex life is good during your menopausal years has a lot more to do with your sex life before menopause, your partner, and your lifelong feelings and interest in sex. Still, hormones do make a difference. In fact, it may be the combination of advancing age; a long-standing, potentially stale relationship; bothersome menopausal symptoms; and declining estrogen levels that creates a perfect storm of sexual discontent.

The Melbourne study found that passage through the menopausal transition was associated with a huge increase in the percentage of women reporting sexual dysfunction. In the early menopause transition, only 42 percent of women had scores indicating sexual dysfunction. Late in the transition, when estradiol levels had significantly declined, 88 percent of women had scores below the cutoff for sexual dysfunction.[16] As women became postmenopausal, they reported less interest in sex, less sexual responsiveness, and more vaginal dryness and pain. Notably, women's feelings toward their partners also became more negative as

192

they passed through menopause.[17]

In the Melbourne study, complaints about menopausal changes included declines in desire, arousal, orgasm, and frequency of sex, as well as pain during sex. As we have already discussed, the reasons for these changes are complex. That said, the study did show that the reduction in sexual function was linked with a decline in estrogen levels.[18] Women who already had mediocre sex lives before menopause were more likely to be pushed toward sexual dysfunction by the hormonal changes of menopause.[19]

So this raises the question of whether taking hormones in a pill or patch can improve your sex life. If the problem is painful sex or bothersome symptoms (nobody wants to cuddle in the midst of a hot flash), then clearly hormones can make a difference in solving the problems that are getting in the way of good sex. But hormones may have a bigger impact on sex than just relief of bothersome menopause symptoms. Hormone therapy may make you want more sex and like it better when you have it.

In a review of the best clinical trials evaluating the effects of menopause hormones on sexual function, researchers concluded that estrogen influences several aspects of sexual function. One study showed that women who used an estrogen patch within 2 years of menopause reported greater satisfaction with sexual activity, sexual fantasies, degree of sexual enjoyment, vaginal lubrication, and frequency of sexual activity.[20] In another study, hormone use increased a woman's sense of sexual attractiveness and led to overall improvements in her sex life.

An Australian study looked at women who had good sex lives and who were happy with their partners. Even though these women didn't have any complaints about their sex lives, things got better with hormone therapy. Women who took estrogen drugs reported increased desire, enjoyment, vaginal lubrication, and orgasmic frequency. Notably, the women who took only estrogen had the most orgasms, followed by the women who took estrogen combined with progestin. Those using only progestin and those in the placebo group had the lowest orgasm scores.[21]

The studies also looked at the role of estrogen therapy in a woman's views of her partner. Unfortunately, estrogen didn't improve a woman's satisfaction with her partner. Even though estrogen may increase desire and arousal, it can't overcome a flawed relationship.

Much of the focus during menopause is on estrogen. But another family of hormones called androgens also may influence a woman's sexual health. Androgens such as testosterone typically are considered male hormones, but they also are found in the female body.

About one-third of circulating testosterone comes from the ovaries, while the remaining two-thirds is created through the conversion of hormone precursors such as dehydroepiandrosterone (DHEA), which are produced by the ovaries and the adrenal glands. This means that the ovaries account for about half of a woman's testosterone.[22] But while menopause dramatically changes a woman's estrogen levels, it doesn't have a big impact on a woman's testosterone levels. The ovary after menopause continues producing testosterone.

Women's testosterone levels do drop off with age, but unlike with estrogen, they don't show a steep decline around the time of menopause. Instead, testosterone levels seem to peak in a woman's thirties, then start falling. By the time she's in her forties, she has about half the level of circulating testosterone as a woman in her twenties. After that, the decline in testosterone slows down.[23] In fact, as women reach menopause, the amount of available testosterone in the body actually increases slightly because other proteins that bind with the hormones start to fall. All this means is that declining testosterone levels probably don't account for the dramatic decline in sexual function after menopause.[24]

Studies trying to link women's sexual problems with testosterone deficiency have been mixed. Several have failed to show any association, while some small studies have linked low testosterone levels with reduced sexual desire and other problems. Part of the problem may be that we just haven't perfected methods for measuring testosterone in women. Many of the studies don't do a great job of measuring sexual function in women, either. Two of the best-designed studies didn't find a connection between testosterone and sexual dysfunction.[25, 26] This doesn't mean there isn't one. It just means we don't entirely understand the role of testosterone as it relates to a woman's sexual health, and you should be wary of any product or practitioner that claims otherwise.

Even though there's still a lot to be learned about natural testosterone in women, researchers have begun to study how testosterone therapy affects a woman's sexual desire and responsiveness. The real question isn't whether a woman's testosterone is considered low or high; what matters is whether using testosterone improves her sexual function.

The North American Menopause Society reviewed 10 studies involving more than 1,500 women that tested testosterone as a treatment for sexual desire disorders. Nine of the studies showed testosterone to be effective in improving sexual desire, arousal, frequency of sexual fantasies, enjoyment, and/or frequency of sex and orgasm. In all but one of the studies, testosterone was given in combination with either estrogen or estrogen and progestin. No data are available about the risks of long-term use.

While the evidence stacks up in favor of testosterone as a potential treatment for sexual arousal problems in women, no product has won FDA approval for this therapeutic purpose. One product, a testosterone patch, had been fast-tracked by the FDA and was considered for approval but was derailed when an FDA panel declined to recommend it. Part of the problem is that the regulatory climate has changed dramatically in the wake of health scares associated with various drugs. Complicating the story is the hormone debate itself and the surprising results of the WHI. It seems clear that any new hormone therapy for women is going to be held to a higher standard in the post–WHI era.

This doesn't mean that testosterone products aren't available to women now. Estratest is a combination estrogen/testosterone drug that is approved for the treatment of menopausal symptoms but is often recommended to treat women's sexual desire problems — an off-label use. Male testosterone drugs have been approved by the FDA, and many doctors prescribe them off-label to women. About one of five testosterone prescriptions is for women.[27] Custom-compounded testosterone drugs are another option; they're available from pharmacists with a doctor's prescription.

Should I Get a Test to Measure My Testosterone?

Most commercially available testosterone tests were designed to measure testosterone levels in men, which are about 10 times higher than in women.[28] The concern is that existing tests aren't sensitive enough to accurately measure the low testosterone levels present in women. In addition, nobody has been able to come up with a defined standard for testosterone deficiency. What may be a low level for one woman might be normal for another.

For this reason, most medical experts don't support testosterone testing to diagnose a sexual function problem. Testing may be useful to monitor a woman's testosterone levels for safety reasons if she is using testosterone therapy, but while some practitioners may measure total testosterone, free testosterone, bioavailable testosterone, or salivary testosterone, the tests aren't considered useful for providing meaningful data about a woman's health. Most doctors will decide whether to prescribe testosterone depending on your symptoms and your answers to questions about your sexual health and history. The only way to find out if testosterone therapy will improve your sexual health is to try it.

What We Don't Know about Testosterone

We know far less about the long-term risks and benefits of testosterone than we do about estrogen and progestin. In its position statement on testosterone therapy, the North American Menopause Society (NAMS) details other potential effects of the hormone.

Bone mineral density. Several small trials

suggest that testosterone added to estrogen therapy improves bone mineral density or seems to reduce bone turnover. No randomized study has looked at the impact of testosterone on fracture risk.

Well-being. One study showed an improvement in well-being among women who had their ovaries removed and used a testosterone patch combined with oral estrogen. Four other studies didn't show any benefit of testosterone over a placebo.

Menopause symptoms. Reliable studies don't show any benefit from testosterone on menopause symptoms.

Lipids. Oral testosterone therapy appears to lower high-density lipoprotein (HDL), the so-called "good" cholesterol, as well as triglycerides in women also taking estrogen. Two studies of testosterone patches showed no change in lipids.

Cardiovascular disease. There aren't enough data from randomized, controlled trials to evaluate the effects of testosterone therapy on cardiovascular disease, including heart attack, stroke, and blood clots.

Cognition. Two small trials showed a slight benefit.

Weight and body composition. Most studies show a tendency toward greater weight gain with testosterone therapy. Two studies showed an increase in lean body mass.

Hirsutism and acne. Facial hair growth and skin problems are potential side effects of testosterone therapy, but most studies show it's not a problem.

Breast cancer. No studies are of sufficient size or duration to evaluate the effects of testosterone on breast cancer. A review of published studies in both animals and humans did not find any link between testosterone therapy and an increase in breast cancer risk.

Since the NAMS review, Harvard researchers have examined data collected from 550 participants in the Nurses' Health Study who were using an estrogen-testosterone combination. The data suggest that these women are at higher risk for breast cancer, but the finding isn't conclusive because of the size of the sample. The overall risk to an individual woman was slight and about the same as for women who use estrogen and progestin.

YOUR HORMONE DECISION

Menopause hormones are an important factor in vaginal and sexual health and should be considered as you make your personal hormone decision. However, it's important to remember that they are only one of several factors that influence your sex life.

Vaginal health is strongly influenced by a woman's estrogen levels, which makes estrogen therapy a reasonable option for women who experience vaginal dryness, itching, or pain. Non-hormone lubricants may be as effective as estrogen. It's also believed that regular sex can improve vaginal health.

For women who feel as though menopause has led to a loss of desire, responsiveness, or other problems related to sexual function, estrogen and testosterone treatments may make a difference. Other treatments, outlined in Chapter 13, also may help. As you discuss these issues with your doctor, it's important to remember that for many women, the answer to their sexual concerns won't come from a pill. The biggest determinant in whether a woman is happy with her sex life during and after menopause is how she felt about her sex life before menopause, as well as how she feels about her partner.

8
HORMONES AND YOUR BRAIN

Women often complain that their menopausal brains just don't seem to work as well as they once did. Doctors say that their menopausal patients often report forgetfulness, a "foggy brain" or fuzzy thinking, memory loss, confusion, depression, struggles with word choice, and other signs of cognitive decline.

Unfortunately, current scientific understanding of the menopausal brain doesn't shed much light on just what's happening physiologically. While women are convinced that their cognitive function during menopause isn't what it used to be, research doesn't always support this. Brain imaging studies do show that big drops in estrogen can produce marked changes in bloodflow to key areas of the brain. While that *might* explain why so many women complain about memory loss during menopause, it's not clear whether the differences that appear in brain scans really translate into a meaningful impact on a woman's everyday life.

Some studies measuring cognitive function during menopause have found no difference among women, regardless of where they are along the menopausal timeline. Some researchers have speculated that the problem isn't menopause but the fact that middle-aged women simply live more-complicated lives than their 20- and 30-year-old counterparts. The constant multitasking, stress, and lack of sleep may be the real culprits taking a toll on our middle-aged brains.

The data on the role of hormones in menopausal brain health are also mixed. Numerous studies have offered conflicting evidence about the impact of menopause and estrogen on brain function, and whether there's anything we can do to improve brain health as we weather menopause and the aging process in general. For years, research has suggested that menopause hormones boost brain health and possibly even prevent Alzheimer's and dementia. But more-recent data from the Women's Health Initiative (WHI) suggest just the opposite — that older women who used menopause hormones had more cognitive problems than women who didn't take hormones.

Hormones also appear to have some connection to depression, sleep quality, and stroke risk. It's all enough to leave your head spinning, but don't worry. As with other areas of hormone research, brain experts are finally beginning to make sense of much of the data. What they are finding is that just as with heart health, there's growing evidence that the timing of hormone use likely makes a difference in brain health as well.

You shouldn't take hormones in the hope of boosting your brainpower; there's simply not enough evidence to show that it makes a difference. But if you've been frightened by headlines linking hormone use with brain problems, keep reading. The evidence shows that women who begin using hormones at the time of menopause to treat symptoms likely face little risk of cognitive problems and may even gain some extra benefit in terms of brain health.

THE AGING BRAIN

Before you can make sense of research into hormones and brain function, it helps to understand a little bit about how your brain ages. Unfortunately, some mental decline due to aging is inevitable. About 10 percent of people age 65 and older have dementia, while many more have some form of mild cognitive impairment. Almost 50 percent of those older than 85 have some form of dementia.[1]

Brain-scan studies show that the brain undergoes physical changes as it ages. Even in healthy individuals, the hippocampus — which plays a crucial role in learning and memory — shrinks over time, as does the brain's ability to process serotonin, a crucial chemical for brain function. "You don't need to be a genius to know that as you get older, your cognition declines," says Declan Murphy, MD, a professor at Kings College in London. "You're not as sharp as you used to be."

Thankfully, the news is not all bad. Research at Harvard University's MacLean Hospital shows that brain development occurs not just in childhood but well into the adult years. A seminal 1994 study looked at 164 normal human brains of various ages from birth to 76, focusing on the formation of the myelin sheath, which is basically the insulation wrapped around the wires of nerve cells to the brain. This process, known as myelination, has a significant impact on the speed of brain function and how quickly one part of the brain myelination can communicate with another part. Depending on what part of the brain it occurs in, it affects not only how quickly you think but also how quickly you act, learn, and process information.

Until the 1994 report, scientists believed that myelination was something that took place during infancy and childhood and stopped after motor and sensory systems were fully developed. But the study found dramatic changes in myelination patterns well into later life. The changes were seen in a part of the hippocampus associated with emotional learning. The study found a 33 percent jump in myelination patterns in the fifth decade and a 55 percent jump in the sixth decade.[2]

Nobody knows exactly what these changes mean, but researchers have speculated that it may explain the emotional maturity of midlife and some of the social behaviors of aging, notes Francine Benes, MD, director of the Harvard Brain Tissue Resource Center at McLean Hospital. For example, it could be the reason that in our forties, we would rather spend quiet evenings with friends than hitting the bars. It could also account for why we typically gain self-confidence as we age. And all that extra brain insulation affects emotions like anxiety, explaining why, as we get older, we no longer sweat the small stuff.

New York University neuropsychologist Elkhonon Goldberg, PhD, has argued that brains get better in certain key ways over time. He concedes that decline in certain areas is inevitable. Memory, concentration, quick thinking, and the ability to learn new things are all hampered by the aging process. But in his book, *The Wisdom Paradox,* Dr. Goldberg notes that there is a shift in the balance of brainpower as we age. The role of the right side of the brain diminishes, and we grow increasingly dependent on the left side.

Aging may take a toll on certain brain functions, but aging and experience reinforce other functions, such as pattern recognition. At its most basic, pattern recognition is what reminds us to avoid a hot stove or to jump back when a car drives through a puddle. But aging helps the brain build up a reservoir of "generic memories" — essentially, the knowledge that can be gained only from life experience. This may be the reason that older people often are better at solving problems or quickly sizing up a situation. And it explains why wisdom and competence increase with age, even as other brain functions begin to falter.

The bottom line: To get wiser, you have to get older.

THE MENOPAUSAL BRAIN

For women, the role of menopause and estrogen in these changes isn't entirely clear. But we do know that estrogen is essential to brain function. The brain is one of the body's most important target tissues for hormones. Estrogen influences brain signaling, affecting the neurotransmitters and receptors that allow brain neurons to communicate with each other. In particular, estrogen appears to stimulate serotonin and norepinephrine receptors in the brain. These are two key brain chemicals linked to cognitive function and memory. Estrogen may also raise levels of another brain chemical, acetylcholine, which can lead to improvements in thinking clarity and memory. And estrogen may work to increase blood flow within the brain, which results in more oxygen and nutrients to brain cells, helping the brain function more efficiently.

Various studies have shown that a woman's cognitive abilities vary depending on where she is in her menstrual cycle, suggesting that our mental dexterity is influenced by estrogen levels throughout our lives. Further evidence that menopause, estrogen, and brain function are inextricably linked comes from brain imaging studies, in which researchers have scanned women's brains at a variety of ages, as they perform challenging mental and memory tasks. Some of this research has compared women taking menopause hormones with those who don't. Consistently, the brain scans show marked declines in brain activity when estrogen is in short supply.

One study from Kings College in London used MRI scans to analyze the brains of 32 women who took the drug lupron, which suppresses ovarian function. The women were given various memory tasks during the scans. The images produced by the MRIs are shocking. In a woman whose ovaries are functioning normally, the image lights up red in areas of the brain related to memory, showing that blood flow is elevated when women are flexing their memory muscles. But in women taking the drug and not producing estrogen, the area associated with memory didn't light up while they were performing the memory tasks. "When we turn off the ovaries, we get significant detriment in terms of memory and accuracy," notes Dr. Murphy. The lighted areas of the scans show that women who aren't producing estrogen have significantly less blood flow in the brain than the women with working ovaries, he says.

Even more troubling are the images taken once the drug is discontinued and the ovaries are switched back on. While most parts of the brain recover — the scans light up red once again — one part in the front of the brain doesn't. The fact that this area doesn't recover once estrogen is lost may explain why many women notice changes in cognitive function during menopause, when estrogen levels are falling.

While estrogen clearly plays a biological role in the brain, whether those changes in the brain scans translate into any meaningful loss in mental ability during menopause remains a matter of debate. Sure, the scans show that estrogen-deprived brains seem to have less action than estrogen-full brains. But does that really make a difference in whether you can find your car keys?

One study, led by researchers at Rush University in Chicago, tried to test the theory that menopause and the corresponding loss of estrogen lead to memory problems.[3] The researchers administered memory and perception tests to 803 women from the Chicago area, ages 42 to 52. The women were part of the large Study of Women's Health Across the Nation

(SWAN), an important government-funded study designed to track the natural history of the menopausal transition.[4]

Most of these women were still approaching menopause — meaning that their natural estrogen and progesterone levels were on the decline, but they hadn't reached the point where their periods had stopped completely. None of the women had used hormone therapy for at least 3 months.

To assess working memory, the researchers instructed the women to repeat backward increasingly long strings of numbers without making a mistake. Another test, this one of perceptual speed, showed the women a series of symbols with corresponding numbers. They were asked to identify as many symbol-number matches as they could in 90 seconds.

To the researchers' surprise, most of the women actually got better with time or at least stayed the same. They didn't get worse. Working memory test scores improved by an average of 3 percent among perimenopausal women. There was no significant change in test scores for postmenopausal women. In the perceptual speed test, women also improved each year, even as their estrogen levels were declining. In this case, however, once the women reached menopause, their scores started to decline slightly.

The news should be reassuring to women, but it's not conclusive. It may be that the women simply learned how to take the tests and got better at it each time. This "learning effect" might have masked any small declines that occurred.

But other studies have also contradicted the notion that menopause is linked to memory problems. The Melbourne Women's Midlife Health Project used memory tests to measure differences in cognitive function during various times of life. Surprisingly, there was no detectable change in memory scores among the menopausal women compared with women of other age groups. Nor was any difference found among women taking estrogen drugs and those not taking the drugs.[5] "I see that as good news," says study author Victor W. Henderson, MD, professor of neurology and neurological sciences at Stanford University. "It means the loss of estrogen, at least in the short run, doesn't affect memory skills."

So how come so many women believe it does? It may simply be that the testing methods scientists use to gauge memory and brain function aren't detecting the subtle changes women themselves notice during menopause. Dr. Henderson also theorizes that women at midlife are facing a range of challenges, not just menopause. Many are managing jobs and households, and menopausal symptoms such as hot flashes and night sweats may be interfering with sleep.

High levels of stress are known to affect memory function. Midlife is a time of tremendous career stress for many women. Their children are graduating from high school and starting college, adding to financial stress. Their aging parents may need extra care or money to pay for medical bills. Rather than menopause, it may be your increasingly complicated life that has left you with a brain that is fatigued and not working as well as it once did.

It's important to note that while problems recalling names and other memory and cognitive complaints are common among menopausal women, few women rate their symptoms as serious.[6] In the SWAN study, about 44 percent of women complained about forgetfulness once they reached the menopausal transition. The number increased slightly to 44.8 percent toward the end of menopause and dropped to 42 percent after menopause. These numbers sound high, but not when you consider that about 31 percent of women in their reproductive years also complained about forgetfulness. Our brains never work as well as we'd like them to, and the problem appears to be only slightly worse during menopause.[7]

HORMONE THERAPY AND THE BRAIN

We know that many women believe that menopause and estrogen loss muddle their thinking and memory. We know that everyone experiences some natural age-related decline in thinking and memory skills. Brain imaging studies have shown that a woman's menopausal experience, natural estrogen, and brain function are inextricably linked. But when women are subjected to memory tests in research studies, no consistent or meaningful differences emerge before, during, or after the menopausal transition. The gap between what women believe and what studies have shown could be explained by flaws in the study design and by the simple fact that it's tough to assess and understand the brain.

Many of the testing methods used by scientists were developed to understand severe cognitive problems. It may be that these tests don't detect the subtle thinking problems that frustrate women. "If you ask the family members or colleagues of these women, very few would say the women are performing poorly," says Hadine Joffe, MD, assistant professor of psychiatry at Harvard Medical School who has conducted brain-scan studies of menopausal women. "There aren't obvious limitations to the world at large, but the women notice that they're working harder to organize things and to get to the same goals."

The bottom line is that most women believe and most doctors accept that whatever the reason, menopause is a challenging time for the brain. So what about menopausal women who use hormones? If losing estrogen might affect memory, does replacing it with estrogen pills improve memory? Most of the evidence suggests that there likely is some cognitive benefit for women who take hormones for the relief of this menopause symptom, but the results are mixed and far from conclusive.

In several laboratory studies, animals given hormone drugs have consistently performed better on memory tests. But women aren't rats or monkeys, and the data on the brain health of women who take hormones aren't as solid. In 2001, the *Journal of the American Medical Association (JAMA)* published a detailed review of the research to date on hormone therapy and cognition in menopausal women. It was a challenging task because all the studies were designed so differently, complicating comparison of their data. The researchers divided their findings into categories describing different areas of cognition. Here's what they found.[8]

Memory. In reviewing studies that examined how hormone use affects memory, the researchers found that most of the data supported the idea that hormone users had better verbal recall than nonusers. Hormone use didn't appear to improve visual memory.

Attention and working memory. Ten studies looked at whether hormone use affects working memory, which is the ability to hold information in the mind, manipulate it, and use it to change behavior without prompting. None of the studies showed that hormone users did better than nonusers in this area. Six studies involved a test requiring subjects to repeat a list of up to eight numbers backward. Only one of these studies found that estrogen users did better than nonusers. Estrogen users typically do better on mental tracking tests, such as arithmetic or repeating the months backward. Two of three studies showed that estrogen use improved a woman's ability to pay attention.

Concept formation and reasoning. In two of three studies measuring the quality of a woman's thinking ability, estrogen users did better on abstract reasoning tests than nonusers.

Motor speed. Reaction time improved in the estrogen users of one study but not in those of a second study. In another study, estrogen users had better clerical speed and accuracy than nonusers.

Verbal function. Only one of four studies found that estrogen users did better than nonusers on tests of language skills. (A more recent study published after the *JAMA* review showed that estrogen users performed significantly better than nonusers on oral reading and verbal memory tasks.[9])

So it was hardly a slam dunk, but estrogen use does appear to make some difference in a woman's cognitive abilities. What was most interesting about the *JAMA* review was its finding that the women who were most likely to show cognitive benefit from hormone use were the same women who were experiencing menopausal symptoms. In four clinical trials where all of the women were experiencing menopausal symptoms such as hot flashes, sleep problems, and fatigue, estrogen use appeared to make at least a small difference. Estrogen use was most likely to improve verbal recall and attention, but mental tracking, concept formation, reasoning, and motor speed were also helped. Equally noteworthy, two trials involving menopausal women who were symptom-free found no improvement in cognitive function.

What does this mean? It's not clear if the estrogen is really helping brain function, or if it is simply relieving tiresome symptoms, allowing women to sleep better and improving their general sense of well-being. The improved quality of life may be the reason that their memory, attention span, and overall brain function is better compared with women who continue to struggle with hot flashes, night sweats, and other menopause symptoms.

Better sleep does improve brain performance. But another theory is that women who are experiencing severe hot flashes are particularly vulnerable to the hormonal fluctuations of menopause, and that their brains show greater effects as well. As a result, women suffering from hot flashes may be more likely to notice cognitive benefits with hormone use.

A Harvard study published after the *JAMA*

review challenges the notion that better sleep is the only means by which hormones improve brain performance. In the study, 52 menopausal women were given a variety of tests to determine their cognitive function level. Then half of the women started using estrogen patches, while the rest used a placebo patch. Three months later, the women were given the tests again. Though there were no meaningful differences in most of the test scores, the researchers did see significant change in one area of complex verbal learning and memory skills.

For this particular test, the tester read aloud a shopping list. After hearing the list, the women moved on to other brain tests. Then 20 minutes later, they were asked to recall and recite the 16-word shopping list. The women taking estrogen did far better on the test, making 43 percent fewer errors after 3 months of treatment. The women in the placebo group made only 9 percent fewer errors.[10] Brain-scan studies of the women confirmed that the estrogen users had greater activation in the parts of the brain associated with complex thinking and decision making.

Notably, the researchers found that a woman's sleeping patterns did not predict cognitive improvement. This suggests that the estrogen was doing more than just helping a woman feel and sleep better. It appears that the hormone was acting directly on the brain, improving mental function.

HORMONES, DEMENTIA, AND ALZHEIMER'S DISEASE

It seems likely that estrogen use does make a difference in a woman's memory and word recall if she's suffering from menopausal symptoms. It's not clear if the estrogen is boosting her brainpower or just helping her stay rested, but in terms of day-to-day life, she probably does feel better.

The bigger question among researchers is whether estrogen use makes a difference in long-term cognitive decline. Does it help stave off dementia and Alzheimer's? Until recently, most research suggested it probably did.

Three important observational studies all strongly suggested that estrogen users are at lower risk for dementia and Alzheimer's. The Manhattan Study of Aging compared 156 postmenopausal estrogen users with 968 nonusers over 5 years. After controlling for variables like education and age, the study showed that estrogen users were 50 percent less likely to develop Alzheimer's disease. And when they did develop Alzheimer's, it started far later in life. The Baltimore Longitudinal Study of Aging followed 230 hormone users and 242 nonusers for up to 16 years. Users were 54 percent less likely to develop Alzheimer's disease than nonusers. Most recently, a study of 1,889 women in Cache County, Utah, showed that those who used hormones had a 41 percent lower risk of Alzheimer's than those who didn't.[11] Two broad analyses of all the data looking at estrogen use and Alzheimer's risk in observational studies showed that hormone users are between 29 and 44 percent less likely to develop the disease than nonusers.[12, 13]

The data are compelling, but as with all observational studies, the question remains whether the hormones really kept these women healthier or if the study was skewed because healthier women were choosing to use hormones. WHI attempted to answer this question with the WHI Memory Study, or WHIMS. The Memory Study tapped into the resources of the WHI, recruiting 7,479 women who were taking estrogen, estrogen and progestin, or a placebo as part of the WHI.[14]

In studying dementia, the researchers faced the same challenges as they did with heart disease. Dementia is a problem that affects older women, so to assess the impact of hormone use on dementia risk in a short period of time, the researchers decided to focus only on older women who were at risk for the problem. While the average age of the women in the WHI was 63 — already far older than the typical hormone user today — the women in the WHIMS trial were even older, ranging from 65 to 79. Given that dementia is a disease of aging, it certainly made sense to study the oldest women. But many researchers now question whether the data are useful to the typical woman in her late forties or fifties who is considering hormone therapy to treat menopausal symptoms.

The data produced by WHIMS are frightening. The women in the study who used hormones had about a 76 percent higher risk of dementia than did nonusers.[15]

Clearing Up the Confusion

Like all things with the WHI, it has taken some time for investigators to be able to make sense of the WHIMS data. Many scientists believe that giving hormones to older women long past menopause was a serious design flaw. Nobody knows exactly why hormone use by older women would trigger a decline in mental function. One theory is that the same clotting effects that caused more heart problems in the WHI's oldest women also may have interfered with blood flow to the brain, leading to mental decline among the women in the WHIMS trial.

Researchers are now working hard to determine whether the timing of hormone therapy makes a difference in risk of dementia and Alzheimer's disease. The data from the Cache County study strongly support this idea and actually fit in nicely with the data generated by WHIMS. The Cache County study is the one that showed a 41 percent decrease in Alzheimer's risk. The women in the study ranged in age from 65 to 102, so like the women in WHIMS, they were older and not representative of the typical woman seeking hormone therapy. But unlike in WHIMS, many of the Cache County women did initiate hormone therapy at the time of menopause to treat their symptoms.

The researchers went back and reanalyzed the data, looking for differences in duration of hormone use. Women in the study who had been using hormones for less than 10 years at the time of the research — suggesting that they started taking hormones later in life and well past menopause — had almost double the risk of dementia, a finding that was strikingly similar to the WHIMS data.

The researchers also identified the women in the Cache County study who were not currently on hormone therapy but had used hormones in the past for 3 years or more. The fact that the women had used hormones but stopped suggests that they had taken the drugs years earlier to relieve menopausal symptoms. These women were 70 to 80 percent less likely to develop dementia.[16] Women in the study who were still using hormones after 10 or more years — suggesting they started taking hormone drugs for menopausal symptoms and never quit — also appeared to be at lower risk, although the data weren't statistically meaningful.

Only a Matter of Time?

Two recent studies add to the evidence that timing of hormone therapy matters, and that hormones taken early in life at the time of menopause — even for short periods — may protect against mental decline later in life.

One of the most interesting studies was conducted by Danish researchers, who looked at 343 women who had taken part in clinical studies of hormones and osteoporosis. These women were ideal because they had taken hormones or a placebo in a controlled research setting. Of these women, 261 didn't continue hormone treatment after the 2- to 3-year study period, while another 82 continued to take hormones. For the women who were on hormone therapy for just 2 to 3 years, the risk of cognitive impairment was 64 percent lower than for women who had never taken hormones. The lower risk was the same for women who had started hormones and stayed on them.[17]

Unfortunately, most of the research to date has looked at hormone use in general, without paying a lot of attention to timing. One of the most important questions raised by the WHI is whether timing matters. Do menopause hormones have a different and potentially protective effect on a woman's brain health when taken close to menopause? And do hormones cause harm, as demonstrated in the WHI, when they are taken late in life long past menopause?

A group of respected menopause researchers attempted to answer these questions in a study called Research into Memory, Brain Function, and Estrogen Replacement, or REMEMBER. In a pilot study of 428 Australian women, the researchers compared early initiators of hormone therapy (those who took it within 5 years of a hysterectomy, or before age 56) with late initiators (those who started hormones later in life and more closely resembled the women in the WHI). Overall, hormone users performed significantly better than nonusers on a test that measured complex cognitive tracking and executive function.

But the most interesting data compared women based on the timing of hormone use. Early initiators scored significantly higher than late initiators on a mental function test and were significantly faster than women who never used hormones on the executive function test. Women in the study between ages 70 and 79 who had used hormones early in life scored significantly higher on a verbal fluency test than women who had never used hormones. And women who started hormones late in life tended to score worse on memory and verbal fluency tests than women who had never used hormones. Overall, early initiation of hormone therapy seemed to have a beneficial effect, while starting hormones late in life seemed to have a detrimental effect.[18]

The Cache County research, the Danish osteoporosis study, and the REMEMBER trial all point in the same direction. All strongly suggest that hormone use at the time of menopause, even for as little as 3 years, lowers the risk of dementia later in life. However, women who start hormones later in life, long past menopause, put themselves at higher risk for mental decline.

HORMONES, MOOD, AND DEPRESSION

Most women have experienced hormone-related mood swings at some point in their lives. For some women, it happens a few days before their periods, when they find themselves in a funk or more weepy than usual. Pregnancy is a time of hormonal highs, while the weeks and months after childbirth are a time when many women experience postpartum depression.

So it's not surprising that hormonal fluctuations associated with the menopausal transition might also result in mood swings, and possibly depression. Doctors regularly report that women come to them with complaints of mood changes during menopause, although scientific studies are inconclusive about the link between menopause and depression.[19] The fact that data from large-scale studies are inconsistent about this link doesn't mean mood changes don't occur. Rather, it likely means that just as PMS and postpartum depression affect only some women, noticeable and severe mood changes probably occur only in some groups of women during menopause.

The Massachusetts Women's Health study found that a history of depression is the best predictor of whether you are vulnerable to depression during menopause. Women who suffered menopause symptoms for more than 2 years before their periods stopped were more likely to experience depression. And women with heavy bleeding or other menstrual irregularities were more likely to experience depression than women with only vasomotor symptoms such as hot flashes.[20]

But several studies now show that perimenopause — the beginning of the menopausal transition when ovarian function starts to decline, periods change, and menopausal symptoms first appear — is the time during which women are most vulnerable to depression.[21] A recent study by Harvard researchers shows that even women without a history of depression are more vulnerable once they enter perimenopause. Overall, the risk of depression doubles once a woman enters perimenopause and may be higher for women with hot flashes and other vasomotor symptoms.[22] A University of Pennsylvania study also showed that women with no history of depression are at risk during the menopausal transition. These researchers found that a woman's risk increases four-fold as she enters perimenopause.[23]

Menopause hormones are effective in improving mood and reducing depression. In a large analysis of 38 studies of hormone therapy and mood, the reviewers concluded that hormone users experienced a 32 percent improvement in mood compared with non-hormone users. Put another way, the average woman who took hormones had a lower level of depressed mood than three-quarters of non-hormone users.[24] While that makes a strong case for using hormones to improve mood and lower depression risk during menopause, it also shows that some women do just fine without treatment. After all, one of four women who didn't take hormones felt just as well as the women who did take hormones. But clearly, for women with severe mood changes during menopause, hormones are one option for evening out the mood swings and avoiding depression.

HORMONES AND SLEEP

Part of the reason so much of the research on menopause and the brain is unclear is because of the effects of sleep — or the lack of it — on thinking and mood. Sleep disturbances are a commonly reported problem among women of all ages, but they increase during menopause. About 31 percent of women in their reproductive years complain of sleep problems; that number jumps to 45 percent 3 years past menopause.[25] Sleep is an important factor for clarity of thinking and overall cognitive function. It also has a big impact on mood and depression.

It's not entirely clear why sleep is a bigger problem for women in the menopausal transition than it is during other times of life. It may be that menopausal symptoms are keeping women awake. Hot flashes, night sweats, vaginal itching, aches, and bleeding problems all may interfere with sleep. Since we know that hot flashes likely stem from brain changes affecting the body's ability to regulate its temperature, it's also plausible that brain functions influencing sleep patterns are affected by declining estrogen levels.

A review of the medical literature found that hormone drugs do appear to improve sleep quality in menopausal women.[26] But how hormones work isn't understood. Although many researchers have speculated that hormones improve sleep quality by relieving menopause symptoms, there probably is more to the story.

German researchers hooked up menopausal women to electroencephalograms (EEGs) to record the electrical activity of their brains. It was a small study of only 11 women, but it nonetheless gives us a glimpse into how hormones might affect sleep. The researchers compared differences in women's sleep patterns while using menopause hormones and while off hormone therapy. Hormone use significantly increased the amount of time that patients were in rapid-eye-movement, or REM, sleep, the later part of the sleep cycle during which dreaming occurs. The researchers also found changes in deep-sleep patterns among hormone users that were similar to the sleep patterns of younger women. While not taking hormones, 10 of the 11 women said they were dissatisfied with their sleep and reported three to five awakenings per night. Once on hormones, 10 of the 11 said their sleep was satisfying, with only one or two awakenings per night.[27]

Not everyone is convinced that hormones make a significant difference in the quality of a woman's sleep. Skeptics were bolstered by reports from the WHI that hormone users in the study didn't experience any meaningful improvements in quality of life, including sleep. The study showed a tiny improvement in sleep after the first year of hormone use, but not much.[28]

While much of the data from the WHI has dramatically improved our understanding of menopause hormones, the data on quality of life changes experienced by hormone users border on ridiculous. Few women in this study had menopausal symptoms. The older women who took hormones didn't get any relief from hot flashes or other symptoms; they just got the side effects. So it's no surprise that their quality of life wasn't improved by taking these drugs. As noted earlier, the WHI wasn't even designed to evaluate the effects of hormone therapy on hot flashes, the single most important quality-of-life issue facing menopausal women.

The WHI quality-of-life assessment did include about 320 women in their fifties who had menopausal symptoms. The group was so small that the data weren't statistically meaningful, but they did show a trend toward improved sleep among hormone users.

Obviously, hormones are not the only way to improve the quality of your sleep. Reducing caffeine and alcohol consumption, treating heartburn, losing weight, and getting regular exercise may all lead to improved sleep quality for women of any age.

Hormones and Stroke Risk

Stroke is a form of cardiovascular disease that affects the arteries leading to and existing within the brain. Strokes can be caused either by a clot obstructing the flow of blood to the brain or by a blood vessel rupturing and preventing blood from reaching the brain.

While most of the early data on hormone use pointed to a protective benefit for cardiovascular disease, the evidence is more mixed in terms of stroke. Some studies have reported no change in risk with hormone use, others have shown a higher risk of stroke among hormone users, and one even suggested a reduction in risk.[29] Some of the studies found no overall increase in risk over time but a higher risk in the first 6 months of use.

As for the WHI, it showed that starting hormones late in life raises the risk of stroke. This likely occurs because hormones are known to increase the risk of blood clots, and blood clots can trigger both heart attack and what's known as ischemic stroke. The WHI found that women who took estrogen and progestin had a 44 percent higher risk of ischemic stroke,[30] while women who used estrogen by itself had a 55 percent higher risk.[31]

It remains an open question whether women who start using hormones at the time of menopause to treat symptoms face the same increase in risk. As we discussed in Chapter 4, WHI researchers have re-analyzed their data and determined that hormone users who were within 10 years of menopause had a lower risk of heart problems than nonusers. The data are less clear for stroke. There were so few cases of stroke in younger women that the data don't have statistical meaning. However, the pattern of higher stroke risk was similar across all age groups.

Don't be alarmed by all the scary-sounding percentages. After all, birth control pills also increase a woman's risk of stroke. For most women, it was a risk they were willing to take during their reproductive years because the likelihood of having a stroke at a young age is so low to start with. What matters most to women considering hormones for the treatment of menopausal symptoms is their absolute risk of stroke. For women under age 65, the risk is extraordinarily low; so even with a marked increase in risk due to hormone use, the overall chance of having a stroke remains very low. A healthy, nonsmoking 55-year-old woman has a 1.1 percent chance of suffering a stroke in the next 10 years. The annual incidence of stroke among women ages 45 to 54 is 0.1 per 1,000 women.[32]

Keep in mind that these numbers are for a healthy woman. If you smoke or have high blood pressure or diabetes, you're at higher risk for stroke to begin with. Your 10-year risk is 6.3 percent, so any increase in that risk due to hormone use becomes far more meaningful.

To get a sense of your personal risk of stroke and how you compare with other people your age, an excellent resource is the Harvard School of Public Health Web site, www.yourdiseaserisk.com. Once you get a sense of your own risk, it should put you one step closer to weighing the risks and benefits of hormones for your personal health situation.

YOUR HORMONE DECISION

The impact of menopause and hormone use on the brain should be a factor as you weigh the risks and benefits of hormones. If you don't have any significant menopause symptoms such as hot flashes or sleep problems, the science shows that hormone drugs probably aren't going to have much of an impact on your thinking and memory. According to studies, women with menopause symptoms may have the most to gain from hormone use in terms of brain health. In the short term, relieving symptoms by taking hormones also may help resolve fuzzy thinking and any other cognitive problems you may be experiencing. But try not to overestimate how much menopause is affecting your cognitive function. Prior to menopause, nearly one-third of women already complain of forgetfulness. And menopause coincides with a highly stressful time in a woman's life.

As you begin coping with menopausal symptoms, be aware that you are likely at higher risk for depression and sleep problems. Both complaints may be helped by hormones or other drug treatments. Some studies show that even short-term hormone use near menopause may lower a woman's long-term risk of dementia and Alzheimer's disease, though the data aren't conclusive. While this potential benefit should give reassurance to women who ultimately decide to take hormones during menopause, women shouldn't take hormones in the hope of lowering their risk of mental decline. There is simply not enough evidence to support this.

While hormone use likely increases stroke risk, if you are a relatively healthy woman under age 65, your starting point for stroke risk already is low. You need to keep this risk in perspective and balance it against the other benefits and risks of menopause hormones as well as your family history of stroke.

Hormones aren't the only option to women for coping with brain issues during menopause. Other treatments, such as antidepressants and sleep aids, can help women affected by symptoms such as mood and sleep changes. An antioxidant-rich diet, stress management, stimulating mental activities like crossword puzzles, and regular physical exercise all can make a big difference in brain function as you get older.

At any age, the main reason people feel as though their memory or thinking skills are slipping is lack of attention, according to Dr. Joffe. Her advice: If something is important, take the time to repeat it and write it down. Make sure that the information is registering in your brain.

9
HORMONES AND
YOUR SKIN

Wrinkles are obviously not a life-threatening health problem. But for most women, the condition of their skin as they get older is an important issue that affects their quality of life. Wrinkles and the quest for more-youthful skin are about more than just vanity. The skin is the largest organ in the body, and it really can be a window into your overall health. Anything that helps or harms the skin could be affecting something else in the body as well.

For years, dermatologists have known that a woman's natural estrogen has a profound impact on her skin. And there's a growing body of research to show that estrogen drugs and creams can make a difference in how skin ages. But the issue of hormones and skin health is largely ignored when women are making the decision whether to use hormones or other treatments during menopause. It's notable that the Women's

Health Initiative (WHI), the biggest-ever clinical trial of menopause hormones, wasn't designed to study the impact of hormone use on hot flashes, vaginal health, or skin aging — all of which are typically the most important concerns of women experiencing menopause.

Because there hasn't been a lot of high-profile research, many doctors dismiss the notion that menopause or the hormones that help women cope with it have any meaningful effect on the skin's appearance. Women themselves are often a little embarrassed about raising the issue of aging skin with their doctors for fear of sounding vain. When a woman talks to her doctor about menopause and hormone therapy, other questions — like breast cancer risk and disruptive hot flashes and sleep problems — seem to trump any worries about skin health.

In the years since the WHI scared many women off menopause hormones, the wrinkle question has resurfaced. Women who stopped taking hormones now complain that their skin seems different. They wonder if their newly discovered wrinkles would ever have appeared had they remained on menopause hormones. It's hard to know the right answer. A lot of time has passed since the summer of 2002; these women are simply older, and so is their skin. Even if they were still taking hormones, chances are their skin would be showing some signs of aging. But several scientific studies support the idea that menopause hormones do offer some protection for aging skin.

MENOPAUSE AND YOUR SKIN

Your skin is composed of two layers. The epidermis is the thin outer layer that consists mostly of cells called keratinocytes. These cells produce keratin, the strong, fibrous protein that is the major component of skin, hair, and nails. The epidermis also contains melanocytes, the cells that produce melanin or skin pigment.

The dermis is the deeper layer that accounts for the bulk of the skin. It's made up of connective tissue and blood vessels. Within the connective tissue are the fibrous proteins collagen and elastin. Elastin fibers make skin elastic and pliable, while collagen fibers plump up the skin and make it strong.

Studies have found that estrogen receptors are present in both layers of skin. For most women, it's certainly not a surprise that hormones play a role in skin health. Whether it was during our teen years, pregnancy, or monthly cycles, most of us have witnessed firsthand how hormonal fluctuations can affect our skin.

But skin aging is driven by a variety of factors. Skin takes a beating from the sun, pollution, smoking, the weather, and other environmental factors. Genetics may be the most important factor. If your mom and dad had wrinkles, chances are you will, too. If your parents had plump, youthful skin well into old age, there are probably fewer wrinkles in your future as well.

After menopause, a woman's skin often reflects the dramatic changes occurring in her body as her natural estrogen declines. When a woman starts to lose estrogen at menopause, her skin becomes less elastic and may be slower to heal. The loss of estrogen also depletes collagen and water in her skin. In fact, collagen declines by as much as 30 percent in the first 5 years after menopause, and it keeps dropping after that.[1] Hyaluronic acid, another important component of skin, declines with age as well.

A woman's bone health may also play a role in her skin health after menopause. We already know that every woman starts to lose bone at a higher rate after menopause. That includes facial bone. It's often overlooked as a cause, but loss of facial bone structure can contribute to wrinkles and sagging skin.

Do Hormone Drugs Make a Difference?

Hormone drugs — whether in pill or patch form, or in facial creams — probably do make a difference in how a woman's skin ages. Several studies show that estrogen use by postmenopausal women increases the collagen content, thickness, and elasticity of their skin.[2] But while changes clearly are happening under the microscope, the big question is whether these changes make a noticeable difference in a woman's appearance.

Let's start by looking at how hormones affect the thickness of a woman's skin. A woman's skin continues to increase in thickness into adulthood. For some women, the thickening may last only until about age 35, but for others, the skin continues to thicken even as late as age 49. Just as with bone, thicker skin is better. Thin skin injures more easily, and because it's less plump, it is more likely to sag or wrinkle.

In 1941, when menopause researcher Fuller Albright, MD, was studying osteoporosis, he noted that postmenopausal women with osteoporosis had skin that was noticeably atrophied.[3] By then, women and cosmetic firms already suspected a link between estrogen and skin health. Before the Cosmetics and Toiletries Act was enacted in the 1930s, estrogen and progesterone creams were sold over the counter and widely used by women to keep their skin looking young. But the new law defined a cosmetic as a product that doesn't alter the structure or function of the skin. As a result, hormone creams were reclassified as drugs and were no longer available over the counter.[4]

Ever since hormone use surged in the 1960s, women and their doctors have speculated that a desirable side effect of using estrogen for menopause symptoms is younger-looking skin. In 1987, researchers were able to demonstrate the link between skin quality and bone health that Dr. Albright had postulated nearly 50 years earlier. They found that in the early years after menopause, skin thickness and collagen content, along with bone mineral density, show steep declines. In particular, skin thickness diminishes by 1.13 percent per year, on average, and collagen levels fall by 2.1 percent — and the drop continues for the next 15 to 18 years.[5]

Several studies conducted in the 1990s show that hormones in pill, patch, or cream form can slow or halt thinning skin and declining collagen levels. In 1992, researchers in Barcelona, Spain, examined skin collagen changes in 194 women, taking skin biopsies from the lower abdominal area. Women using hormones in pills or skin patches showed an increase in skin collagen content ranging from nearly 2 to 5 percent over the 12-month study period. The women who didn't use hormones, meanwhile, posted declines in collagen levels.

Because so many factors — including environmental pollution, smoking, and sun exposure — can influence skin health, a group of Canadian researchers decided to study a group of nuns to better isolate the effect of estrogen on the skin. Nuns make a good study group because they tend to have similar lifestyles, eat the same foods, and not smoke, so any potential benefit of hormone use is easier to measure. In the Canadian study, 60 postmenopausal nuns were given either estrogen pills or a placebo. Doctors examined the skin around the thigh area using ultrasound and skin biopsy. The thighs of the nuns taking estrogen had measurably thicker skin than those of the nuns who didn't take estrogen.[6]

Another important study confirmed that estrogen didn't just maintain skin thickness but actually improved it. In 2001, London researchers used ultrasound technology to measure skin thickness in the forearms of 84 women. Some of the women were younger and hadn't yet reached menopause (or started taking hormones), while others were in the midst of the menopausal transition.[7] The study showed that the women who were using menopause hormones had about double the skin thickness of the women who weren't using hormones. But what was really surprising about the data was that the hormone users had nearly the same skin thickness as the younger women who hadn't yet reached menopause. This benefit occurred regardless of how long the women had been on hormone therapy, whether 6 months or 6 years. The finding supported earlier studies suggesting that the collagen benefit occurs after about 6 months of hormone use; after that, hormone therapy simply halts collagen loss.

Of course, most aging women aren't all that worried about the quality of the skin on their arms, stomachs, or thighs. What they really care about is how aging shows up in their faces. Most studies look at other body parts because it's easier, and because there's no risk of facial scarring if bits of skin have to be removed for testing. But a

2003 study looked directly at the impact of estradiol cream on the face. The women applied the estradiol cream to one side of their faces and a placebo cream to the other side. Skin biopsies showed the epidermal skin to be 23 percent thicker on the hormone side than on the placebo side.[8]

Another way researchers have gauged the impact of hormones on a woman's skin is to look at elasticity. A loss of elasticity can cause skin to sag. Just as with skin thickness, several studies have shown that hormone use makes skin more elastic and pliable. Women who use estrogen drugs maintain their skin elasticity, and some even see improvement. By comparison, the non-hormone users in these studies lose skin elasticity as they age.

WHAT ABOUT WRINKLES?

While the impact of estrogen on skin thickness and elasticity is well documented, the more important question is whether those changes result in a noticeable difference in a woman's appearance. In short, does using estrogen help prevent wrinkles?

Though there's not a lot of research looking at the link between estrogen use and wrinkles, the available data do strongly suggest a benefit. An important 1997 observational study, the first National Health and Nutrition Examination Survey (NHANES I), assessed the skin health of 3,400 postmenopausal women over age 40. Women who used estrogen were 24 percent less likely to have dry skin and 32 percent less likely to have wrinkles.[9] In 1998, Barcelona researchers enlisted 730 women to help determine how hormone use and smoking affected wrinkle risk. Their study confirmed the NHANES data showing that estrogen use influences wrinkle risk. In the study, lifelong nonsmokers who took hormones had fewer wrinkles than nonsmokers who didn't take hormones. Another key piece of information from this study is the fact that estrogen use didn't make a difference in wrinkling of smokers.[10] Estrogen, with all its potential for keeping skin young looking, can't work miracles by overcoming the ravages of a damaging behavior like smoking.

But observational studies always raise the question of the healthy user effect. That is, does hormone use really reduce wrinkles? Or are women who use hormones healthier to start with and less likely to engage in behaviors that harm skin, such as smoking and excessive sun exposure? The sparse evidence from clinical trials to date does seem to support what the observational

248

studies show — that estrogen use really does lower wrinkle risk.

In 1994, French researchers compared the effects of estrogen cream and a placebo in 54 postmenopausal women. After 6 months, estrogen was significantly more effective than the placebo in improving fine wrinkles.[11]

In 1996, a study from Vienna, Austria, suggested that estrogen creams could actually reverse signs of skin aging in women prior to menopause. It measured the effects of estrogen creams on 59 premenopausal women. After 6 months of treatment, wrinkle depth had decreased by 61 to 100 percent — meaning that in some cases, the wrinkles disappeared completely.[12]

While these numbers sound impressive, they are far from conclusive. The Vienna study didn't have a placebo group, meaning that all the women used estrogen cream. The problem is that skin quality improves when you take care of it. These women were paying more attention to their skin and rubbing cream on it every night. It's impossible to know whether it was the extra skin care or the estrogen that made such an impact on their skin health.

More recently, Yale researchers tackled the question of estrogen and wrinkles. Theirs was a small study, looking at only 20 women.[13] However, it's the only blinded study to gauge the effects of oral estrogen on wrinkles. This is important because wrinkles are judged by people, so it's easy for bias to creep in. The researchers in the Yale study didn't know whether a woman was using estrogen or a placebo, adding credibility to their findings. They also used a widely accepted wrinkle scoring system, as well as a special device that measures skin hardening.

All the women in the study were at least 5 years past menopause. Of the 20 women, 11 had never used menopause hormones, while 9 were longtime hormone users. The women were comparable in terms of age, race, sun exposure, sunscreen use, and smoking history. They were evaluated for wrinkles in 11 different parts of the face, including frown lines, cheek and neck folds, and eye wrinkles. To avoid subjective scoring variations, the women were evaluated by only one plastic surgeon who wasn't aware of whether they had ever used hormones. When the wrinkle scores were tallied, the scores of the non-hormone users were 50 percent worse than those of the hormone users.

The researchers also conducted a more

objective test measuring skin rigidity. Softer, more pliable skin has more collagen and is less likely to wrinkle. Again, the non-hormone users were 50 percent worse in their forehead measurements and 2 1/2 times worse in their cheek measurements.

While the study is too small to be conclusive, it supports what many women and doctors have believed for years: Taking estrogen at the onset of menopause has a significant effect on a woman's skin and appearance. "I have long believed that I can tell by looking at a postmenopausal woman whether she is receiving hormone therapy," says University of Miami dermatologist Leslie Baumann, MD.[14]

The fact that the Yale study showed a skin benefit in longtime users also fits with the notion that the timing of hormone therapy may make a difference in whether it's beneficial or risky to a woman's health. Some studies have failed to show a skin benefit from hormone use, but the reason may be that the studies showing no effect involved older women.[15]

The Kronos Early Estrogen Prevention Study (KEEPS) will attempt to answer the question about whether the timing of hormone use makes a difference in the risks and benefits of hormones. As part of that research, the Yale doctors plan to continue studying the effects of menopause hormones on skin quality.

CREAMS VERSUS PILLS AND PATCHES

After reading about the estrogen and skin research, you may be tempted to rush out and buy some estrogen cream to rub on your face. Unfortunately, the answer isn't that simple. Although some drug companies make estrogen creams for vaginal health, no prescription hormone creams have been approved by the FDA for skincare. Some doctors may prescribe a vaginal cream for facial skin care, but it's not widely used for that purpose.

Most doctors say it's not a good idea to start using estrogen cream directly on your face. There are not enough data about how facial skin absorbs the estrogen and any potential side effects or risks. We do know that estrogen creams and gels are absorbed through the skin and into the bloodstream. So women with a uterus have to be careful about using topical estrogens because they still may face a higher risk of uterine cancer.

In addition, most of the studies of menopause hormones show that you get pretty much the same skin effects whether you take estrogen by pill, patch, or cream. Right now, no estrogen product makes any claims about skin health. Drug companies have done extensive research in this area, but none of the evidence has been conclusive enough to convince the FDA that hormones boost skin health.

Your Hormone Decision

Nobody believes that women should take menopause hormones simply to avoid wrinkles. But many doctors believe that skin protection is one potential benefit that women should consider as they weigh all the benefits and risks of hormone therapy. Only you can decide how much of a factor wrinkles and facial aging should be in your overall hormone decision. Many doctors believe that how you feel about your appearance can have a profound impact on your overall health and habits.

In a recent medical journal article, Wake Forest University dermatologist Zoe Diana Draelos, MD, noted that any assessment of the risks and benefits of hormone therapy needs to include a discussion of skin health. She noted that problem skin can lead to depression, which is an important risk factor in a woman's cardiovascular health. She also raised the issue of whether a woman who has fewer wrinkles and feels good about her appearance might exercise more frequently, possibly further offsetting some of the risks associated with hormone use.[16]

The issue is particularly relevant to women who are worried about their bone health. If you are at high risk for low bone density and osteoporosis (as outlined in Chapter 6), your risk of wrinkles also might be higher. There's a strong correlation between skin thickness, collagen content, and bone mineral density in postmenopausal women, and women with osteoporosis are at higher risk for thin skin.[17]

Once you've assessed your bone and skin health, it's important to remember that estrogen loss is only one factor in how your skin ages. Think about your mother and grandmother. Did they wrinkle? Did they use hormones? Factor in your lifetime sun exposure. Did you spend hours cooking in baby oil at the beach, or did you slather on the sunblock? What's your smoking history? Do you eat lots of fruits and vegetables and exercise regularly? Do you take care of your skin? Are you willing to consider plastic surgery or Botox injections to reduce wrinkles? All these questions will help you determine how much weight you should give to your skin health and appearance when you are making your personal hormone decision.

Estrogen can't undo a lifetime of bad skin habits. However, there are other options for taking care of your skin and looking younger as you age. Given how hard it's been for scientists to prove that estrogen helps your skin, any benefit — if there is one — is likely to be modest. At best, estrogen may help slow skin aging, but it won't stop it. Every year you get older, your skin gets older, too.

10
HORMONES AND
OTHER BODY PARTS

Menopause hormones clearly will help relieve the hot flashes, night sweats, sleep problems, and vaginal changes associated with the menopausal transition. By now, it should be clear to you that hormones — both natural and in pills, patches, or creams — have a far-reaching impact throughout your body. The effects of hormones on a woman's cardiovascular, breast, and brain health have gotten the most attention in recent years, but there is a far bigger story to tell. Hormones influence a woman's health from head to toe. Until you have a sense of all the ways hormones work and act in your body, you can't fully weigh all the risks and benefits of hormone use.

Here's a summary of other body parts and functions that appear to be influenced by menopause hormones.

Colorectal cancer is the third most common cancer in women, after breast cancer and lung cancer. A woman's chance of developing colon cancer in her lifetime is 1 in 18. By comparison, her chance of developing breast cancer is 1 in 8. Colon cancer also accounts for 10 percent of the more than 273,560 cancer deaths expected to occur among women in 2006. (For the same year, an estimated 15 percent of cancer deaths will be due to breast cancer.[1]) A woman's risk of colon cancer jumps once she turns 50, which is about the same time in life she is coping with menopause symptoms and making a decision about hormone use.

While much of the attention to hormones and cancer has focused on breast cancer, the colon cancer story is a surprising one. In observational studies, the risk of colon cancer is almost 50 percent lower among estrogen users than among non-estrogen users. Research also shows a link between the use of birth control pills and a lower risk of colon cancer.

Data from the Women's Health Initiative (WHI) support the notion that menopause hormone users are less likely to develop colon cancer. Among women in the WHI, the risk of colon cancer was 44 percent lower for those taking estrogen and progestin than for those not using hormone therapy.[2] Researchers noted that the death rates from colon cancer were the same for both groups, but that hormone users were more likely to be diagnosed at a more advanced stage. This probably doesn't mean that menopause hormones cause more-aggressive cancers. Rather, there were simply fewer new cancers among hormone users. The data on advanced cancers were slightly skewed because so few early cancers were found at all.

Unfortunately, the data from the estrogen-only segment of the WHI are less clear, which may have something to do with the fact that so many women stopped taking hormones during the study period. There was no statistically meaningful difference in colon cancer risk between estrogen users and nonusers.

Scientists don't really know why menopause hormones might lower colon cancer risk. One theory is that high levels of certain digestive compounds can increase risk, and hormones tend to lower levels of those chemicals.

Only you can determine how much the potential colon cancer benefit should factor into your decision about hormone use. It is a benefit that is often ignored when doctors advise women about the risks and benefits of hormone drugs.

HORMONES AND THE OVARIES

The hormone story as it relates to ovarian cancer is confusing. That's because most women have been told that if they use birth control pills — which contain higher levels of estrogen and progestin than menopause hormones — they will dramatically lower their risk of ovarian cancer. This is likely due to the fact that the risk of ovarian cancer increases the more you ovulate. Women who use hormonal forms of birth control stop ovulation, so they stop the monthly cellular destruction and repair process that can trigger a cancerous mistake in their ovaries.

Once a woman reaches menopause, ovulation stops on its own. It's less clear how taking hormones at this point in life affects a woman's risk of ovarian cancer. The scientific data are all over the map. One analysis of 15 studies concluded that estrogen therapy does not increase risk,[3] while another analysis of 9 studies showed a higher risk among hormone users.[4] In a major study of more than 44,000 women, those who used estrogen only — particularly for 10 or more years — were at significantly increased risk for ovarian cancer. However, the study didn't find any increased risk among women who used estrogen and progestin.[5]

The problem with much of the data on menopause hormones and ovarian cancer risk is that ovarian cancer is so rare. There are just too few cases from which to draw meaningful conclusions. In the WHI, there was no statistically significant difference in ovarian cancer risk among hormone users and nonusers. There was a trend toward higher risk in the hormone group; however, it could very well be due to chance.

It's difficult to advise women about menopause hormones and ovarian cancer risk. Ovarian cancer is considered a relatively rare disease; at the same time, there's no suitable screening method for it, and it is particularly deadly because it's typically caught so late. To keep perspective, consider that ovarian cancer is the eighth most common cancer among women, after breast, lung, colon, and uterine cancer, non-Hodgkin's lymphoma, melanoma, and thyroid cancer. It's the fifth most common cancer killer among women, accounting for 6 percent of female cancer deaths — the same as pancreatic cancer.

The data on hormone use and ovarian cancer risk are far from conclusive, but they do strongly suggest that hormones increase risk. Even if that's the case, the disease is so rare that a woman's overall risk remains exceedingly low, unless she has a pronounced family history of the disease.

HORMONES AND THE UTERUS

Uterine cancer is the fourth most common cancer among women. The good news is, it is highly treatable. It accounts for only 3 percent of cancer deaths among women.

It's been clearly established that using estrogen by itself sharply increases the risk of cancer of the endometrium, which is the uterine lining. Women who've undergone a hysterectomy needn't worry about this risk because they no longer have a uterus. Women who still have a uterus and who want to use hormones are advised to take progestin to prevent the risky buildup of the uterine lining that can trigger precancerous changes.

There is some suggestion that women who use both estrogen and progestin have a lower overall risk of uterine cancer than non-hormone users. The WHI showed a 19 percent decrease in uterine cancer risk among estrogen and progestin users. The data didn't reach statistical significance, so the finding could be due to chance. However, the general direction of the data toward lower risk should be reassuring to women who ultimately choose to use hormones.

HORMONES AND THE BLADDER

The female body has estrogen receptors throughout the urogenital area. Just as the vagina is markedly affected by the loss of estrogen during menopause, so are other organs, muscles, and body parts along the urogenital tract. But like so many issues with menopause hormones, the hormone and bladder story is confusing.

Bladder-control problems are common as women age. One issue is that women who have had children have experienced more wear-and-tear on the bladder. Aging further weakens muscles, which allows the bladder to slip. It appears that declining estrogen levels during menopause can cause further weakening of these muscles. Estrogen loss also can affect the lining of the bladder and urethra, which — just like the vagina — needs the hormone to stay plump and healthy.

Numerous studies have suggested that

estrogen therapy can improve or cure incontinence as women age. It may be particularly helpful for urge incontinence, which is the inability to control urination long enough to make it to the bathroom.[6] In another type of incontinence, called stress incontinence, small amounts of urine leak out when a woman sneezes, coughs, or laughs. Most reports have concluded that estrogen therapy isn't effective for stress incontinence.[7]

The WHI has raised questions about whether estrogen therapy is a good idea for women with any kind of bladder-control problem. In both WHI hormone studies, women who used hormones appeared to have a higher risk of developing or aggravating bladder-control problems.[8] Of course, as we have discussed throughout this book, we need to be careful about how we interpret the WHI data. There are several concerns about the incontinence data. One is that incontinence appeared at far higher rates among women in the WHI than in the general population, suggesting that it may have been overdiagnosed. Also, the WHI primarily involved older women, and many of the incontinence problems occurred mainly in older women — again suggesting that estrogen therapy affects the body differently when taken years after menopause compared with at the onset of menopause. Other potential flaws with the WHI data include the high dropout rate and the fact that women with certain side effects may have been treated differently by study doctors, thus skewing the study results.

These and other problems have caused some researchers to question just how meaningful the incontinence data really are. An editorial in the *Journal of the American Medical Association* cited many of these concerns, concluding that the WHI is an important study but that far more research is needed to fully understand the impact of hormones on incontinence after menopause.[9]

So how do you factor this information into your hormone decision? For women coping with menopause, it's important to know that questions have been raised about the role of estrogen therapy in bladder-control problems. Women shouldn't take estrogen just to solve bladder problems. If you are a woman with menopausal symptoms, and you have a bladder-control problem, estrogen use may improve bladder control — or worsen it. You should simply be aware that bladder problems are associated with aging and that several new non-hormonal drugs are available to help treat them.

Some studies have linked estrogen use with a lower risk of urinary tract infections. It may be that estrogen helps the body resist infection by lowering vaginal pH levels and preventing bacteria from thriving in the vagina. It's not clear if women get this benefit from oral estrogen therapy. The studies to date suggest that estrogen creams and estrogen-releasing rings may have the biggest impact on lowering a woman's risk of urinary tract infections.

HORMONES AND THE GALLBLADDER

The gallbladder is a small, pear-shaped organ that is situated behind the liver. Its job is to store bile, which helps with the digestion of fat.

Gallbladder disease is more common in women than in men. Gallstones are solid stones that form in the gallbladder. They are made from cholesterol, bile salts, and calcium. Gallstones occur in 10 to 20 percent of the population over age 40, but only a fraction of those people develop symptoms. Among the symptoms of gallbladder disease are mild to severe pain after eating, nausea, fever, and jaundice.

The risk of gallbladder disease rises among women who have relatives with gallstones, those who are obese, and those who have high cholesterol or certain intestinal diseases such as Crohn's or ulcerative colitis. Using estrogen, either in birth control pills or in menopause hormones, is also associated with a higher risk of gallbladder disease. Several studies have shown that women who take menopause hormones are at increased risk for gallbladder disease.[10, 11] For example, women in the Nurses' Health Study who used estrogen were nearly three times as likely to undergo a gallbladder operation as non-hormone users. And as expected, hormone users in the WHI had a higher risk of gallbladder problems than did nonusers.

Typically, when someone develops gallbladder symptoms, the recommended treatment is removal of the gallbladder — a minimally invasive procedure.

HORMONES AND BODY FAT

There is a general belief among women and even some doctors that menopause hormones contribute to weight gain. The scientific data simply do not support this.

Both women and men are prone to weight gain in midlife. It may be because of lifestyle changes, increasing stress, or just a general decline in physical activity. Whatever the reason, the research shows that in women, weight gain is not related to hormone use.

In a large clinical trial called the Women's Health, Osteoporosis, Progestin, Estrogen (Women's HOPE) study, researchers tracked 2,673 healthy postmenopausal women for a year. The women took varying levels of menopause hormones or a placebo. Everybody in the study put on weight, but the women taking hormones actually gained less than the women in the placebo group.[12]

In the WHI, there was a small but significant change in weight after the first year of the study. A higher proportion of women in the hormone group lost weight compared with those taking the placebo.[13]

HORMONES AND BLOOD PRESSURE

Blood pressure is another area in which a woman's natural hormones seem to offer some protective effect before menopause. Studies show that women have significantly lower blood pressure than men from puberty to menopause, the time frame in life when a woman's natural estrogen levels are at their highest. However, following menopause, a woman's blood pressure tends to rise until it is in roughly the same range as the blood pressure of men of the same age. This pattern is similar to what happens to a woman's heart attack risk before and after menopause. Notably, after menopause, women also become more sensitive than men to the hypertensive effects of sodium.

All of this leads to the question of how hormone drugs might affect blood pressure. In theory, if a loss of estrogen is linked with an increase in blood pressure, then adding estrogen in pill or patch form should help lower blood pressure. Some studies do show that when hormones are given to postmenopausal women, they lead to lower blood pressure both at rest and during exercise. Hormone therapy also appears to enhance the heart's ability to regulate blood pressure.[14]

However, these are short-term treatments. It still is not clear whether long-term estrogen use results in a consistent reduction in a woman's blood pressure. A review of the medical literature on estrogen and blood pressure turns up mixed results. Some studies show a benefit, some show a partial change, and some show no impact at all. In one study, only nighttime blood pressure readings declined as a result of estrogen therapy. This may be important, because elevated blood pressure at night has a strong correlation to the risk of developing hypertension.[15]

The evidence to date strongly suggests that estrogen — both natural and in drug form — influences blood pressure. It may be that its impact is greatest in certain women at risk for hypertension and that its effect is modest or negligible in other women.

HORMONES AND YOUR ACHING BODY

When a woman approaches menopause, her mother, her doctor, and her friends will talk at length about hot flashes, mood changes, irregular bleeding, and vaginal health. But there is little discussion about the fact that common menopause symptoms include body aches, stiffness, and pain. A Swedish study of nearly 4,000 women estimated the incidence of body pain to be between 50 and 70 percent among menopausal women, depending on their age.[16] Another recent study found that women with lower levels of natural estrogen were more likely to develop arthritis of the knee.[17]

Treatment with menopause hormones appears to offer some relief from body pain, although it's not entirely clear why this is so. The WHI was not designed to measure the effectiveness of hormones in treating menopausal symptoms; nevertheless, some data were collected from the small number of women in the study who complained of symptoms. Joint pain and stiffness, general aches and pains, and lower back and neck pain weren't as common among the women in the WHI compared with women in other studies. In the WHI, between 10 and 25 percent of women complained of pain, with the variation depending on the specific pain symptom and the woman's age. The WHI did show that treatment with estrogen and progestin resulted in a 25 percent improvement in general aches and pains and a 43 percent reduction in joint pain and stiffness.[18]

HORMONES AND DIABETES

One of the most neglected areas of menopause hormone research is the role of hormones in diabetes. Type 2 diabetes is the most common form of diabetes and usually is triggered by a combination of obesity, poor diet, lack of exercise, and genetics. The body becomes unable to effectively process insulin and can't make enough of the hormone to maintain normal blood-glucose levels. (In type 1 diabetes, the pancreas doesn't produce enough insulin. It is most common in children and young adults, and unlike type 2, it isn't preventable.)

Insulin is important because it promotes the storage and use of all nutrients, including sugar. Once full-blown diabetes occurs, glucose is barricaded from cells and instead accumulates in the bloodstream.

How diabetes damages the body isn't entirely understood. One theory is that all the excess sugar in the bloodstream triggers a process similar to rusting. The sugar begins to stick to things, damaging kidneys, blood vessels, and nerves.

While it is true that people with diabetes can make diet and lifestyle changes to manage their illness fairly well, complications from the disease can be tragic. The leading cause of death among people with diabetes is heart attack and stroke, and about 40 percent of all heart attacks are caused by diabetes. Diabetes is also the leading cause of blindness, kidney failure, impotence, and amputations. It even shortens life expectancy by 5 to 7 years.

Given the far-reaching impact of diabetes as a public health issue, it's surprising that some of the most telling data about menopause hormones and diabetes have been virtually ignored. In the WHI, estrogen and progestin users were 21 percent less likely to develop diabetes, while estrogen-only users were 12 percent less likely to develop the disease. The earlier HERS trial (the Heart and Estrogen/Progestin Replacement Study) showed that the combination of estrogen and progestin reduced the risk of diabetes by 35 percent. Major observational studies have also found a lower risk of diabetes among women who take menopause hormones.[19]

As a health issue, diabetes is clearly as important as cardiovascular disease, breast cancer, and stroke, yet it doesn't resonate as such with the public. For reasons that aren't clear, the role of menopause hormones in reducing the incidence of diabetes has been largely ignored in the hormone debate.

■ ■ ■ ■

PART THREE:
MAKING YOUR OWN
CHOICES

■ ■ ■ ■

11
THE PROGESTIN QUESTION

The more we have learned about menopause hormones over the years, the more we've become aware of two very different hormone stories taking shape. There's one for the women who use estrogen by itself, and another for the women who must use a combination of estrogen and progestin. Unfortunately, for many women who opt for hormone therapy, progestin is a necessary evil. But once you learn more about it, you likely can find ways to minimize your exposure to it.

You probably already know why some women take estrogen and some take a combination hormone. Women who still have a uterus when they begin the menopausal transition and who opt for hormone therapy are advised to take a combination of estrogen and progestin. Estrogen causes a buildup of the endometrium, which is the tissue that lines the uterus. This buildup dramatically increases a woman's risk of uterine cancer. But if she uses progestin along with estrogen, her risk of this cancer drops dramatically. Depending on the timing of progestin, the hormone prevents the thickening of the endometrial lining or causes it to slough off much like a period. Women who have undergone a hysterectomy — which is the surgical removal of the uterus — have the option to take only estrogen.

The problem is, most of the unpleasant side effects of menopause hormone use are triggered by the progestin, not the estrogen. Irregular bleeding and breast tenderness are the most common, and these side effects are the main reason women stop hormone therapy. Progestin can also act as a diuretic and affect the smooth muscle in the bowel, causing bloating and constipation. Bruce Ettinger, MD, clinical professor of medicine and radiology at the University of California, San Francisco, says he tells women that progestin is "the hormone that's not going to make them feel better."

In the wake of the Women's Health Initiative (WHI), new questions have been raised as to whether progestin does more than cause unwanted side effects. What has become increasingly clear is that there may be additional risks and benefits of taking a combination of estrogen and progestin compared with taking estrogen by itself. For all the inherent flaws in the WHI, perhaps one of its most important contributions has been to highlight the fact that progestin may be a more important factor in the risks and benefits of menopause hormones than previously thought. While it clearly protects the uterus, it also may have a significant impact on blood clotting, breast cancer risk, heart and brain health, and symptom relief.

If you don't have a uterus, you don't need to take progestin for any reason. But you still might want to read this chapter to learn more about this important hormone. Becoming familiar with the potential side effects and risks of progestin will help you understand why many of the biggest worries about menopause hormones likely don't apply to women who take estrogen alone. Learning more about progestin will help you determine which risks of hormone use you really need to think about and which risks don't apply to you.

If you haven't had a hysterectomy and are considering menopause hormones, the progestin question is an important part of your decision. If you choose to take menopause hormones, you really don't have a choice about whether to take progestin. But you do have options. Increasingly, doctors are debating whether the type of progestin makes a difference in risk. And there are several ways of taking progestin that may influence your symptoms and bleeding patterns, as well as minimize your long-term risks. Although there are still many questions to be answered, the existing science should help you make the most informed decision possible.

WHAT IS PROGESTIN?

In discussions of menopause hormones, you will come across various terms to describe the "other" important female hormone. Doctors and patients alike tend to use the terms *progesterone, progestin,* and *progestogens* interchangeably. *Progesterone* is the actual hormone made inside a woman's body by her ovaries and adrenal glands and by the placenta if she is pregnant. *Progesterone drugs* have the same chemical structure as the progesterone made by the body. You will often hear these drugs called "natural progesterone," but this is misleading. A progesterone drug does match the chemical structure of progesterone made by the body, but it's still a man-made drug. There's nothing natural about it. A *progestin* is a man-made hormone that works pretty much like the progesterone made by the body. In other words, progestin seeks out the same hormone receptors as progesterone and acts on the body in a similar fashion. The progesterone made by the body, as well as the progesterone and progestin made by drug firms and pharmacists, are all *progestogens.*

A woman's natural progesterone is essential to the reproductive process and promotes gestation — which, incidentally, is how it got its name. A woman's progesterone levels rise and fall during her monthly menstrual cycle. Progesterone works by preparing the uterus for implantation of the egg. If an egg isn't fertilized, progesterone levels drop sharply, causing the uterine lining to shed and resulting in a period. After menopause, a woman's natural progesterone virtually disappears, although small amounts are still produced by the adrenal glands.

Progestins and progesterone drugs can be used alone or in combination as birth control pills. Sometimes, they're prescribed to prevent miscarriage. Progestins can be used in the "morning after" pill to prevent a pregnancy. And, of course, they are prescribed during menopause to lessen the impact of estrogen on the uterus.

Progestogens are complex, with the potential to act on three different types of hormone receptors in the body. They can act on progesterone receptors; they can "down regulate" estrogen receptors, which essentially means that they counteract the effects of estrogen; or they can act on androgen receptors. The fact that progestogens have so many different actions helps explain the range of possible side effects, which vary depending on what type of progestin or progesterone drug you use.

How Do Progesterone and Progestin Treatments Affect the Uterus?

The main benefit of progestin and progesterone drugs is to lower a woman's risk of uterine cancer (also called endometrial cancer, after the endometrium that lines the uterus). For years, it was believed that taking progestin in combination with estrogen simply canceled out the negative impact of estrogen on the uterus. But more-recent evidence suggests that progestin may actually go a step further, giving women who use estrogen and progestin hormones added protection against uterine cancer compared with women who don't use hormones at all. The Million Women Study in Britain showed that combination hormone users had a 23 percent lower risk of uterine cancer than women who didn't take any menopause hormones. Progestin not only reduces the number of estrogen receptors in the uterus, it also converts estradiol to a less potent form of estrogen called estrone.

While the uterine benefit is reassuring, most women aren't at high risk for uterine cancer to start with, so this shouldn't be a huge factor in your hormone decision. A Swedish study found that fewer than 1 in 200,000 women get uterine cancer before age 50. After 50, the incidence jumps to about 6 cases per 100,000 women; after 60, it increases to between 7 and 8 cases per 100,000 women.[1] (By comparison, the annual incidence of breast cancer is about 129 cases per 100,000 women.[2])

A woman who uses estrogen without progestin is about five times more likely to develop uterine cancer. That said, several other factors besides estrogen use also can increase a woman's risk. Most of them relate to the amount of natural estrogen a woman's body is exposed to over her lifetime. Here are some of the other factors that influence a woman's risk of uterine cancer.

Total number of menstrual cycles. The more

menstrual cycles you have in your lifetime, the higher your risk. So if you started your period before age 12, or if you have a very late menopause, your risk may be higher. If you started your period earlier and experience menopause earlier, your risk likely isn't different from that of women who started their periods in their teens.

History of infertility or never having a child. Pregnancy increases progesterone, so many pregnancies will lower risk, while never being pregnant raises risk.

Family history. Uterine cancer can run in families. A condition called hereditary non-polyposis colon cancer can increase a woman's risk of uterine cancer by as much as 60 percent. If you have several family members with colon cancer or uterine cancer, you might consider genetic testing to see if you also are at risk.

Obesity. Having a lot of fat tissue increases a woman's natural estrogen levels and may cause a five-fold rise in her risk of uterine cancer.

Diabetes. Uterine cancer may be four times more common in women with diabetes than in women without. The link may be obesity, because people who are overweight are at higher risk for diabetes. There is some evidence that diabetes not linked to obesity also raises the risk of uterine cancer.

Other risk factors. Using the drug tamoxifen, having a history of breast or ovarian cancer or ovarian disease, or receiving radiation therapy in the pelvic area may increase the risk of uterine cancer.

WHAT ELSE DOES PROGESTIN DO?

When doctors first started prescribing progestin to women who were taking estrogen for menopause symptoms, very little thought or research went into the practice. The thinking was that it was a good way to protect the uterus from the deleterious effects of estrogen. Clearly, it is. But what didn't enter into the treatment equation is the fact that the body has estrogen and progestin receptors all over, which means that the impact of progestin treatment isn't isolated to the uterus. Research shows that progestin likely has effects on the brain, heart, breasts, colon and urogenital tract, among other tissues.

Here's a look at the potential role of progestin in symptoms and other factors associated with menopause.

Progestin and hot flashes. There has been some suggestion that progestin works to reduce hot flashes. Unfortunately, the data aren't conclusive. Some of the early studies used high doses of progestin, which did appear to have a benefit; today, however, progestin is taken at a relatively low dose. Another study funded by a menopause hormone manufacturer found some added benefit from standard doses of progestin in relieving hot flashes. But a closer look at the study shows that the number of women who reported improvement was small, and not everyone believes the data are reliable. It appears that the benefit of progestin for most women is, at best, borderline. There's no solid evidence that low doses of the hormone provide any meaningful relief from hot flashes compared with what estrogen does by itself. On the other hand, adding progestin doesn't interfere with estrogen's ability to relieve hot flashes, either.

Progestin and the brain. Progestin can have a powerful effect on the brain; sometimes, it is prescribed to women with epilepsy to treat the disorder. Progestin is known to increase endorphins and can cause sleepiness and mood changes. That's why many doctors advise women to take their progestin at night to minimize the impact of these side effects. Some animal studies have suggested that while estrogen appears to help the brain, progestin may cause harm. In one study, researchers who mimicked a stroke injury in rat brains found that treating the rats with progestin worsened the injury.[3]

Progestin and the heart. Studies have shown that progestin may lessen some of the heart-protective benefits of estrogen. While researchers are still debating whether estrogen actually does protect the heart, there is lots of evidence that estrogen leads to important changes in risk factors related to heart health. For instance, the hormone raises high-density lipoprotein (HDL), the good cholesterol. But in an important study called Postmenopausal Estrogen/Progestin Interventions (PEPI), it was shown that women who took estrogen alone got bigger boosts in HDL than women who took a combination of estrogen and progestin.[4]

Another study called Estrogen Replacement on Progression of Coronary Artery Atherosclerosis (ERA) found that while estrogen increased levels of a substance known as C-reactive protein (CRP), a risk factor for heart disease, adding progestin resulted in even larger rises in CRP.[5] Importantly, the study noted that just because the hormones raised CRP levels, it didn't produce any meaningful changes in the women's health. Their heart disease didn't get worse because of the higher CRP score. Still, these findings are important because they show that progestin does have a different impact — albeit one we don't quite understand — on the markers for heart disease compared with estrogen alone.

Progestin and the bones. The data here are mixed. Some studies have shown that progestin does not result in any additional benefits to the bones in women who are using estrogen. Other studies have identified slight increases in bone density with the addition of progestin to hormone therapy. Even if there is a benefit, the effect is only slight and shouldn't be a significant consideration as you are weighing the risks and benefits of combination hormones.

Progestin and the breasts. When doctors first started prescribing progestin, the belief was that because the hormone blocked the effects of estrogen on the uterus, it would have similar positive effects in the breasts. But most of the evidence suggests that progestin acts very differently above the waist than below it. Studies in animals, particularly monkeys, show that progestin actually increases cell proliferation in the breasts.[6] (Cell proliferation is an increase in cell growth and cell division, which can lead to the cellular mistakes that trigger cancer.)

In one small observational study of 86 postmenopausal women, the combination of estrogen and progestin triggered more cell proliferation in the breasts than did estrogen by itself.[7] And in a finding that may help explain some of the differences we've seen in breast cancer risk among estrogen-only users and combined estrogen/progestin users, the same study showed that the cellular proliferation triggered by progestin was focused in the part of the breast where most cancers develop.

We also know that progestin users often experience breast tenderness and dense mammograms. Most studies that have examined mammographic density show that a far greater percentage of women taking combination estrogen and progestin have increases in breast tissue density than women on estrogen alone.[8]

While increased cell proliferation and greater breast tissue density are associated with cancer risk, questions remain about the real role of progestin in breast cancer. The WHI data, while far from conclusive, also point an accusing finger at progestin more than estrogen. In the two WHI hormone studies, women taking a combination of estrogen and progestin had a higher risk of breast cancer than non-hormone users. However, women who were taking only estrogen, without progestin, had a lower risk of breast cancer than non-hormone users. Based on these findings, estrogen appeared to protect the breasts, while estrogen and progestin appeared to increase breast cancer risk.

From a scientific standpoint, it's tricky to compare the two arms of the WHI to each other. The health of the women in the two groups was very different, so numerous other factors — including obesity rates among women in the study — could have influenced the results. That said, the difference is so striking that many researchers believe much more study is needed to better understand the impact of both estrogen and progestin on the breasts.

DOES THE TYPE OF PROGESTIN MATTER?

There are so few data comparing different progestin regimens that nobody knows with scientific certainty whether the type of progestin makes a difference in side effects, risks, and benefits. But a growing number of doctors believe the real problem isn't the combination of estrogen and progestin. The culprit, in their opinion, is the type of progestin that has been widely used in studies. It's called medroxyprogesterone acetate, or MPA. It's the same progestin in the birth control drug Depo Provera and the combination menopause hormone drug Prempro.

Historically, MPA has been the most commonly used progestin. Much of this was simply convenience, as it was the main combination therapy available to women and the one with which doctors had the most experience. However, there are other combination drugs on the market that include the progestins norethindrone acetate, norgestimate, levonorgestrel, and drospirenone, which also are the active ingredients in popular birth control pills. Another option is micronized progesterone, sold under the brand name Prometrium. It is made from wild yams and soy and has the same chemical structure as the progesterone made in a woman's body.

There's very little research comparing different progestins. A major study called the Million Women Study is one of the few research efforts to evaluate the use of estrogen in combination with various types of progestins. The study recruited 1,084,110 British women between ages 50 and 64 who were getting mammograms on a regular basis. Not surprisingly, women who used estrogen and progestin were at higher risk for breast cancer than non-hormone users. The risk of breast cancer wasn't affected by the type of progestin. Women in the study who were on medroxyprogesterone acetate, norethisterone, or norgestrel all faced about the same risk. This surprised a lot of people who expected to see differences in MPA compared with the other progestins. Most researchers now interpret these data as showing that synthetic progestins are about the same in terms of their effects on the breasts.

Unfortunately, this important study didn't compare the progestins to micronized progesterone, a compound that is chemically identical to the hormone made by a woman's body. The PEPI trial examined the differences between MPA and micronized progesterone. While there are not a lot of data from which to draw major conclusions, the PEPI study did show that there are at least minor differences in the effects of micronized progesterone on the body compared with MPA. Progesterone appears to be less potent than MPA, and as a result, progesterone was less likely to dampen the positive effects of estrogen than MPA was.

For instance, in the case of HDL, estrogen alone raised this good cholesterol more than combination estrogen and progestin. However, women who took micronized progesterone experienced bigger jumps in HDL than women who took MPA. The PEPI study also showed that using MPA raised blood sugar, suggesting that MPA may aggravate a diabetic tendency more than micronized progesterone will.[9] In terms of breast health, there were differences, but they weren't huge. In the PEPI study, 19.4 percent of women who used estrogen and a low dose of MPA showed increased tissue density in their breasts, a risk for breast cancer. Among women using micronized progesterone, 16.4 percent of women had increased tissue density.

Recently, University of South Florida researchers tried to compare the different effects of micronized progesterone and MPA using a novel imaging technique to observe bloodflow, blood vessel structure, and activities of various blood cells in a live animal. After the researchers administered a dose of MPA to laboratory rats, the animals showed visible signs of brain blood-vessel damage, inflammation, blood clot formation, and impeded blood flow. Using the same techniques, the research team determined that micronized progesterone did not cause similar vascular toxicity.

Whether any of these differences translates into any meaningful changes in a woman's overall health risks isn't clear. But the observation that micronized progesterone might have fewer negative effects than MPA, along with the troubling data emerging from the WHI about progestins generally, has prompted many doctors to promote the use of micronized progesterone instead of MPA.

So why wouldn't every doctor recommend it? Part of it has to do with experience. Progestins have been around a lot longer, and most of the available data about progestin use are based on MPA so women who use it have to take two pills or combine patches and pills. For women who prefer a single combination pill, the only option is to take a pill with MPA or another synthetic progestin. Also, micronized progesterone isn't sold in a combination pill with estrogen.

Prometrium, the only FDA-approved micronized progesterone brand, is suspended in peanut oil, so women with peanut allergies can't take the drug. Another option is to go to a compounding pharmacist, who can custom-mix a peanut-free version of micronized progesterone.

Continuous, Cyclic, or a Few Times a Year? Reducing the Risks of Progestin

While the type of progestin is one part of your hormone decision, you also need to consider how often you want to take it.

Most doctors today prescribe a continuous dose of progestin along with estrogen. Taking a continuous dose should eliminate periods altogether and resolve irregular bleeding. The problem is that in the first 6 months or possibly even a year of use, spotting and irregular bleeding may still occur, an issue that frustrates many women so much that they eventually stop their menopause hormones altogether.

Another option is to take cyclic progestin therapy. This is similar to how many women use progestin in birth control pills. It involves taking estrogen for a few weeks, then adding in progestin. When you stop the progestin, the lining of the uterus sheds, just like a monthly period.

Though most women prefer continuous treatment, some studies have suggested that cyclic therapy might be slightly less risky than continuous progestin use. The largest study to date — the Million Women Study, with more than 9,000 cases of breast cancer — didn't show any differences in risk among women based on the number of days a month they used progestin. In the PEPI study, changes in breast tissue density were about the same among cyclic and continuous hormone users. In a Swedish study, about 28 percent of women on combined/

continuous hormone therapy showed changes in breast tissue density compared with 10 percent on cyclic therapy.[10] Another study involving 175 women found increased tissue density in the mammographies of 52 percent of women receiving combined/continuous estrogen and progestin therapy, but only 13 percent of those on the cyclic regimen.[11]

So there is some evidence to suggest that cyclic therapy — which gives a woman a regular period — is slightly less risky than continuous therapy, which ideally stops periods altogether. But one of the best things about menopause is no more periods, which is why many women don't like the idea of cyclic therapy and ongoing periods, even if the risk is slightly different.

Taking Less Progestin
There are other options beyond continuous or monthly cyclic progestin. Some doctors are bucking the conventional wisdom and beginning to offer women who still have a uterus a seldom-talked-about option: taking little or no progestin at all. In a seismic shift in thinking, some doctors are now prescribing a dose of progestin just once or twice a year; some are opting to eliminate it entirely.

At one time, the idea of giving estrogen

alone to women who haven't had a hysterectomy would have been unthinkable because of the risks of uterine cancer. Steven R. Goldstein, MD, professor of obstetrics and gynecology at New York University School of Medicine, has been a vocal supporter of "long-cycle therapy," which involves reducing or possibly eliminating the progestin dose. Dr. Goldstein says it's possible to give a woman just one or two progestin doses a year or to eventually eliminate progestin entirely if she is monitored with transvaginal ultrasound to detect simple hyperplasia, a benign condition that occurs when the uterine lining grows too much. Although hyperplasia can be a precursor to uterine cancer, in most women, the problem is easily treated with a dose of progestin to slough off the uterine lining.

Not everyone agrees with Dr. Goldstein's methods. For some women, occasional doses of progestin and ultrasound monitoring may not be practical. Taking progestin every 6 or 12 months may trigger a heavy, uncomfortable bleeding episode that can last for 2 weeks. And regular monitoring with transvaginal ultrasound is expensive. It can cost $250 or more and often it isn't covered by insurance.

Another solution may be to reduce the

estrogen dose so much that it no longer causes a buildup of the uterine lining, making regular monitoring or occasional progestin doses unnecessary. One study from the University of Connecticut looked at low-dose estrogen in 167 women, half of whom took 0.25 milligram — one quarter of the standard dose — of micronized estradiol, which is similar to a woman's natural estrogen. Those women were given micronized progesterone just twice a year during the 3-year study, and they didn't show any increase in hyperplasia or uterine cancer.[12]

In a manufacturer-sponsored study of a very low-dose estrogen patch, women using the patch didn't take progestin for 2 years, but didn't show any increased risk of endometrial problems.[13] The very low doses of estrogen appear to protect against osteoporosis, but it's not clear whether they would have a meaningful impact on other menopause symptoms, such as hot flashes or vaginal atrophy.

Other Options

For women who don't want to try long-cycle therapy, there are other options for limiting progestin exposure. A vaginal or intrauterine progestin may be a good way of directing the progestin to the uterus where it's needed and avoiding side effects in the rest of the body. Progesterone creams rubbed into the skin might also be an option, but there are limited data on how much of the hormone is absorbed into the body. Some studies have shown that a 3 percent cream rubbed in twice a day does the trick, but you really need to talk to your doctor about how he or she plans to monitor the health of your uterus if you are using a progesterone cream. If the cream isn't potent enough, your body won't absorb enough to protect the uterus.

In the end, women who try one of these alternative approaches to progestin should be prepared to invest a little extra time and effort to keep the uterus healthy. Some doctors use transvaginal ultrasound monitoring to make sure that the uterine lining isn't building up. Others simply check in regularly to make sure that their patients are not having irregular bleeding, a sign that there may be an unwanted thickening of the uterine lining.

Taking an unconventional approach to progestin requires a bigger commitment. Given that there has been far more study of traditional continuous-cycle progestins, many women and their doctors choose traditional therapy because it's convenient and relatively predictable.

YOUR HORMONE DECISION

One of the great benefits of the recent science on menopause hormones is that it has prompted women and their doctors to think a lot more about the "other hormone" involved in hormone therapy. So much of the emphasis is on the risks and benefits of estrogen because it's the hormone that will relieve your symptoms. But progestin is an important part of your hormone decision. If you have a uterus and decide to take hormones for the relief of menopause symptoms, here is a summary of your progestin options.

Take a combination estrogen/progestin pill in a continuous dose. It is convenient and the most-studied way of using combination hormone therapy. The downside is that you might experience irregular bleeding, breast tenderness, bloating, and constipation. It's unclear just how much progestin changes the risks and benefits of estrogen use. Most of the data point to the fact that progestin probably blunts some of the protective effects of estrogen and slightly increases certain risks compared with estrogen alone, particularly in terms of breast cancer. Nonetheless, your overall risk of a health problem resulting from estrogen and progestin use during menopause remains low, particularly if you limit your use to less than 5 years.

Take estrogen plus progestin in a cyclic dose a few days a month. This isn't all that different from the way you may have used birth control pills during your reproductive years. You will continue to have monthly periods. The main advantage is that you will know every month that your uterine lining has shed, lowering your risk of uterine cancer. There is some limited evidence that taking cyclic therapy poses a slightly lower risk than continuous progestin therapy. The main disadvantage is that you will continue to have periods.

Switch to micronized progesterone. Many doctors are advising their patients to use either continuous or cyclic treatment with estrogen and micronized progesterone rather than any of the various progestins that are widely available. The advantage is that micronized progesterone, which is made from yams and soy, is chemically identical to the progesterone made by your body. There is limited evidence that micronized progesterone has slightly fewer negative effects than traditional progestin, but the data are far from conclusive.

One negative is that there is only one FDA-approved micronized progesterone, and it isn't available as a combination drug. This means you will have to take separate estrogen and progesterone pills, which may be less convenient. The other issue is that progesterone is suspended in peanut oil, so if you have a peanut allergy, you can't take the commercially prepared version. You have the option of getting your progesterone from a compounding pharmacist, but you need to seek out a reliable and experienced compounder.

Consider long-cycle therapy. Instead of taking progestogens every day or a few days each month, consider taking them every 3 months or 6 months or once a year, depending on your doctor's advice. If your doctor supports this option, the advantage is that you are dramatically reducing your progestin exposure. The downside is that doctors remain divided on how long it's safe for a woman with a uterus to go without progestin. If you pursue this option, be prepared to undergo regular monitoring to make sure your uterus remains healthy.

Consider vaginal or uterine progestin. This directs the progestin to where it's most needed without the risky side effects in the rest of the body. The downside is that many

300

women would rather take a pill than a vaginal treatment, and there hasn't been a lot of study on this type of progestin.

The best advice I've heard from doctors about progestin has to do with how you start taking it. Many doctors simply hand women a prescription for a combination hormone drug with the instruction to start taking it for the relief of menopause symptoms and to check back to report how they feel. The women might notice improvement in their hot flashes with the estrogen, but they also may experience breast tenderness and irregular bleeding — at which point they may question whether hormones are really worth the trouble.

But some doctors suggest that every woman begin hormone therapy by taking just the estrogen by itself for the first several weeks, even if she still has a uterus. The practice isn't considered risky if done for only a short time, and taking estrogen by itself will give you a better idea of what the hormone will do for you and how much symptom relief you will experience.

Once you get a sense of whether estrogen is relieving your hot flashes, minimizing any sleep disturbances, or improving your vaginal health, you're ready to add in the progestin. Most of the worst side effects of hormone therapy come with progestin use. By starting the hormone later, you will have a better sense of which side effects are from the estrogen and which are from the progestin. If estrogen by itself makes you feel a lot better, then any side effects or frustrations you experience with progestin may be worth it. If you don't notice much of a difference with estrogen, then you shouldn't expect any more benefits when you add progestin to the mix.

Your doctor may increase your dose of estrogen if you're not getting any benefit from a lower dose. But remember, increasing the estrogen dose requires an increase in the progestin dose — and the more progestin you are taking, the more side effects you will experience. The bottom line is that as you weigh the risks and benefits of menopause hormones, you should talk with your doctor about all your options in hormone therapy, including the different types of progestin and their different methods of delivery.

12
PRESCRIPTION HORMONES: PILLS, PATCHES, CREAMS, AND RINGS

If you have made the decision to take menopause hormones, your next step is to consider what kind you want to take. You have a number of different hormone preparations to choose from, and they can be delivered to your body in different ways. Hormones come in pills and patches as well as creams and gels that are rubbed onto the skin or inserted into the vagina. Hormones can be implanted beneath the skin or inserted as vaginal or intrauterine rings. There are brand-name hormone drugs, generic therapies, and custom-mixed prescription hormones made by a compounding pharmacist.

With so many options, choosing which hormone preparation to take can be daunting. Chances are your doctor has his or her own opinions about what the best choice is. Among medical researchers, there's a lot of debate about which formulation or type of hormone is safest. The main question is whether women should use the same types of hormones studied in the Women's Health Initiative (WHI) or whether they should choose different forms of estrogen and progestin in the hope of avoiding the risks identified in the WHI. You will hear arguments for both viewpoints. According to the FDA, we should assume that all hormones carry the same risks and benefits as those studied in the WHI. We don't have any solid evidence that any one type of hormone is better or worse than another.

An important study that supports this view is the Million Women Study, which involved one million British women over age 50. Unlike the WHI, in which all the women used either conjugated equine estrogen by itself or with medroxyprogesterone or a placebo, the women in the Million Women Study used a variety of hormone products administered as pills, patches, or implants under the skin. Surprisingly to medical experts, there was little or no difference in the risks and benefits observed among the different forms of estrogen or progestin being used.[1]

These results, coupled with the lack of any evidence to the contrary, suggest that the most conservative and practical approach is to assume that all hormones pose the same benefits and risks to your heart, bones, breasts, and other body parts. As we have seen throughout this book, the risks of hormone therapy to the typical woman seeking relief from hot flashes and other menopause symptoms are relatively low.

Even though we really don't know whether one type of hormone is safer or better than another, there are many reasons that women might choose different products. Some simply feel better using one type of estrogen or progestin compared with another. Others prefer the convenience of a patch or want to focus their treatment on vaginal health, so they opt for a vaginal cream. The good news is that women have more options and more information about menopause hormones than at any other time in history.

Estrogen Pills

Conjugated equine estrogens (Premarin, Prempro, Premphase). These hormone drugs are made from a mix of estrogens derived from horse urine. Premarin is for women who are using only estrogen, while Prempro and Premphase are combination pills that also contain progestin. Premarin and Prempro were the hormone drugs used in the WHI. Because Premarin and Prempro have

305

been the most-prescribed menopause hormones over the years, the vast majority of scientific data on hormone therapy are based on these drugs.

Premarin is a complex drug, and scientists still don't fully understand all of its components. So far, they have identified 10 distinct estrogen compounds, as well other biologically active steroids. The primary compounds are estrone sulfate, constituting approximately 53 percent of the estrogens; and equilin sulfate, accounting for about 25 percent of the product.[2]

Premarin is derived from the urine of pregnant mares. This may sound a little gross, but animals aren't a particularly unusual source for ingredients in drugs, cosmetics, and supplements. For years, insulin was produced from the pancreas of pigs or cows, while the blood-clotting drug heparin is derived from animal organs. Even the collagen that is injected into people's lips and faces to erase wrinkles comes from the connective tissue of pigs or cows.

Once the urine is collected from mares, it's processed at a Canadian facility where it undergoes an extraction and purification process that involves hundreds of steps. By the end, no urine is left — only a complex mixture of estrogens and some androgens.

The hormones are blended with other inactive ingredients to form a tablet or cream.

The medical community is divided about Premarin. Some doctors swear by it, while others prefer to prescribe estrogens that are more chemically similar to a woman's natural estrogen. The advantage of Premarin is that we know more about it than any other hormone. In fact, one concern about switching to other forms of estrogen is that some of the potential benefits of hormone therapy may not be realized if the unique combination of hormones present in Premarin isn't used.

One example is breast health. In the WHI, women who took only Premarin appeared to get some protection against breast cancer. This was surprising, given that many breast cancers are estrogen-based. What isn't clear is whether there is something unique about Premarin's unusual mix of hormones that conferred extra protection. One WHI researcher speculated that the androgens present in Premarin might have played a role in the breast cancer results. We simply don't know the answer.

In the end, it comes down to personal choice. Some women feel great on Premarin, while others switch to a simple estrogen because of side effects. For women who use a combination of estrogen and progestin, Prempro is particularly convenient because it's available as a pill that contains both hormones.

Plant-based conjugated estrogens (Cenestin, Enjuvia). These drugs are made from a mixture of several estrogens derived from plants. Cenestin has nine estrogen compounds, while Enjuvia contains 10 estrogens that the manufacturer claims are chemically similar to the estrogens found in Premarin. The downside of Cenestin is that no long-term clinical trials have been performed, though it has received FDA approval for short-term use. Enjuvia is a new product, so the data on it are limited.

In general, most studies show that all oral estrogens result in the same circulating blood levels of estrogen, so there's no real advantage or disadvantage to choosing one form over another. On an individual basis, some women may experience more symptom relief or more side effects with one form than another.

One reason to take conjugated estrogens may be convenience. They typically have a longer half-life than other oral estrogens, which means you may end up taking fewer pills.

Esterified estrogens (Estratab, Menest,

Estratest). Esterified estrogens are a mixture of synthetic estrogens. They contain approximately 80 percent estrone sulfate and approximately 11 percent equilin sulfate.[3] Clinical comparisons of esterified estrogens and conjugated equine estrogens are limited to a single crossover trial that reported significantly better short-term cognitive function and depression scores among menopausal women while they were taking esterified estrogens compared with conjugated equine estrogens.[4] A more recent study suggests that esterified estrogens carry a lower risk of blood clots than conjugated equine estrogens.[5] More study is needed to confirm these findings.

17-beta estradiol (Estrace, Gynodiol, Activella, generic estradiol). Estradiol is a chemical match to the dominant form of natural estrogen produced in a woman's body before menopause. There's no evidence that it's better or safer than other estrogens, but many women like the idea of taking a chemically identical drug. Although estradiol is not as well studied as conjugated equine estrogens, there is still plenty of research to document its safety and effectiveness. The Million Women Study, which involved many women taking estradiol, found no differences in the health benefits and risks compared with women taking other forms of estrogen.

In terms of convenience, users of oral estradiol may need to take it twice a day rather than once a day. The biggest advantage is that unlike the conjugated estrogen products, estradiol comes in a generic form, which is cheaper than brand-name estrogens.

Estropipate (Ogen, Ortho-Est, generic estropipate). This is a synthetic estrogen compound, which means it acts like an estrogen in the body but is chemically different from any naturally occurring estrogen.

Ethinyl estradiol (Femhrt, Estinyl). This synthetic estrogen is typically found in birth control pills but sometimes serves as a menopause hormone.

Estradiol acetate (Femtrace). A synthetic estrogen, estradiol acetate converts to estradiol once it's in the body.

HORMONE PATCHES

Estrogen patches (Alora, Climara, Estraderm, Vivelle, Vivelle Dot, Menostar, estradiol patch). Increasingly, many doctors are prescribing patch hormones to help women cope with menopause symptoms. The main advantage of patch treatments is that a woman can take a lower dose than if she uses estrogen in a pill form. This is because estrogen, when swallowed as a pill, has to pass through the liver before it reaches estrogen-sensitive tissues. Liver enzymes inactivate some of the estrogen, so only a portion of a dose is actually used to relieve menopausal symptoms. With a patch, the hormones are absorbed directly into the bloodstream, and as a result, a woman can get symptom relief with a lower dose of estrogen.

Another potential benefit of the patch is that it carries a lower risk of blood clots. The risk is lower because it's the passage of estrogen through the liver that increases risk. The biggest downside of the patch is that it's a patch — it's visible on the body, it gets kind of dirty toward the end of the week, and it has to be changed. But many women find changing patch treatments once or twice a week easier than remembering to take a daily pill.

The main differences between patches are how they look (some are small and clear, while others are large and flesh-colored) and how often they need to be changed (either once or twice a week). Most patches contain estradiol. One patch, Menostar, contains a low dose of estradiol. It's prescribed for the treatment of osteoporosis; whether it also offers relief from menopause symptoms remains to be seen. Unlike the other patch treatments, which require progestin for women who have a uterus, Menostar has such a low dose of estrogen that women typically require only occasional doses of progestin if they still have a uterus.

Combination patches (Climara Pro, Combipatch). These patches contain a combination of estrogen and progestin. They are convenient for women with a uterus who want a patch treatment but don't want to take an oral progestin as well.

PROGESTOGENS

Medroxyprogesterone acetate (Provera, Prempro, Premphase, Amen, Cycrin). MPA is the most commonly prescribed progestin. It's a synthetic hormone, which means it isn't a chemical match for natural progesterone, but it nonetheless acts like a progestin inside the body. Like Premarin among estrogens, MPA is probably the most-studied progestin. But many doctors and patients find that it is too potent and causes too many side effects.

The WHI has raised a lot of questions about the safety of MPA and whether progestin — and MPA in particular — may be the culprit in the range of health problems experienced by older women using hormones. In the WHI, women taking estrogen alone didn't have a higher risk of heart attack or breast cancer, while women who took estrogen plus MPA did. As a result, many doctors are looking at other forms of progestin for women who still have a uterus.

The main benefit of MPA is convenience. Combined with Premarin, it forms Prempro, which requires taking just one pill a day.

Megestrol acetate (Megace). This progestin usually is used in the treatment of cancer and endometriosis but often is viewed as too potent for menopausal women who are also taking estrogen.

Micronized progesterone (Prochieve vaginal gel, Prometrium). Many doctors say that micronized progesterone is a better option for hormone users because it typically causes fewer side effects. The downside is that the oral form is not packaged as a combination drug, so women who use it must take at least two pills a day. Another concern is that it's suspended in peanut oil, which means that women with nut allergies can't use the brand-name progesterone product, although they can go to a pharmacist for a custom-compounded progesterone drug.

A common side effect of micronized progesterone is sleepiness, which is why doctors may advise women to take the hormone at night. If drowsiness becomes too much of a problem, it may prompt some women to switch to a different progestogen.

Other synthetic progestins. Several synthetic progestins typically found in birth control pills are sometimes used in menopause treatments. These include norgestimate (Ortho-Prefest), norethindrone acetate (Femhrt, Activella, Combipatch), and levonorgestrel (Climara Pro).

COMBINATION HORMONE PRODUCTS

Continuous combined (pills: Prempro, Femhrt, Activella, Angeliq; patches: CombiPatch, Climara Pro). A continuous combined pill or patch provides a dose of estrogen and progestin every day. The continuous dose of progestin means that you won't get monthly withdrawal bleeds; however, many women do experience unpredictable spotting, which usually stops within 6 months of starting treatment. Continuous combined products offer various combinations of estrogen and progestin. One relatively new drug, Angeliq, uses the progestin drospirenone, which is unusual in that it reportedly is less likely to cause water retention and bloating than other combination products.

Cyclic combined (Premphase). The only cyclic combination product, Premphase contains the same hormones as Prempro. The only difference is that the pills containing progestin are taken only the last 10 to 14 days of the month. Although a menopausal woman is no longer fertile, using a cyclic regimen will create a monthly cycle similar to her period. (For a discussion of the advantages and disadvantages of cyclic therapy versus continuous therapy, see Chapter 11.)

Intermittent combined (Ortho-Prefest). Instead of taking progestin every day or for the last half of the month, as with continuous and cyclic regimens, a woman who's using intermittent therapy takes progestin in cycles of three days on and three days off. It's not well studied, but the idea is to give the body regular breaks from progestin to lessen side effects while providing enough progestin to prevent periods.

Esterified estrogens/testosterone (Estratest). A combination of estrogen and testosterone may be prescribed for the relief of hot flashes and other menopause symptoms in women who don't get relief from estrogen alone. Although Estratest is not approved for the treatment of sexual dysfunction problems associated with menopause, some doctors still recommend it for this purpose.

Because so few women use Estratest compared with other estrogen products, there are little data on its risks and benefits. A recent review of data from the Nurses' Health Study showed that women who used Estratest were at slightly higher risk for breast cancer than women who used combination estrogen and progestin.[6] However, most of that risk showed up in the first few years of treatment and dropped after 5 years of treatment — suggesting that rather than causing cancer, the drug may simply make existing cancer show up sooner.

VAGINAL HORMONES

Vaginal creams (Estrace, Premarin, Cenestin, Estinyl, Menest, Ogen, Ortho-Dienestrol). Vaginal creams help restore vaginal tissue, relieving vaginal dryness, itching, burning, and irritation caused by the loss of natural estrogen. The creams are highly effective in treating menopausal symptoms, but they can be messy.

Vaginal rings (Estring, Femring). Femring is a flexible ring that women can insert into the vagina much like a tampon. One dose lasts for 3 months. Most women find the ring comfortable and say that it doesn't interfere with sex and isn't felt by their partner. Femring is a systemic estrogen, meaning that it treats hot flashes and other menopause symptoms. Women with a uterus who use Femring also need to take a progestin to prevent a risky buildup of the uterine lining.

Estring is a low-dose vaginal ring, also used for 3 months. It helps treat vaginal and urogenital issues associated with menopause. It has a much lower dose of estrogen than Femring, and as a result, women who still have a uterus may be allowed to take only an occasional dose of progestin.

Vaginal tablets (Vagifem). These estrogen tablets help restore vaginal health. They come preloaded into a single-use applicator. They are inserted daily for 2 weeks, then typically just twice a week after that.

HORMONES FROM YOUR PHARMACIST: THE "BIO-IDENTICAL" DEBATE

Chances are you've already heard about so-called "natural" or "bio-identical" menopause hormones. When people use these terms, they are usually talking about compounded hormones.

Compounded hormones have surged in popularity as a result of the book *The Sexy*

Years, written by former sitcom star Suzanne Somers. Unfortunately, women have been left with the impression that compounded hormones are better and safer than commercial hormone products. Many women believe compounded hormone products aren't drugs — or for that matter, aren't even hormones. This simply isn't true. Compounded hormones are still hormones. They are made from the same or similar bulk ingredients that pharmaceutical companies use to make their products. The difference is that they are mixed by your local pharmacist rather than produced on a large scale by a big manufacturer. They also are packaged differently than commercial hormone preparations.

Compounding pharmacies play an important role in the health-care system. Pharmacists prepare custom-mixed drugs for patients who for some reason can't use commercial drugs manufactured by pharmaceutical companies. For instance, compounders might make a chewable tablet or a dye-free version of a particular medicine for a patient with special needs. Many patients who have allergies to certain drug ingredients, or who want medications no longer manufactured on a large scale, turn to compounders to provide treatments that they may not be able to get anywhere else.

Ever since the results of the WHI were announced, compounding pharmacies have played an increasingly important role in menopause treatment. Compounded hormones have a different chemical structure than the hormones studied in the WHI, so many doctors, pharmacists, and women are touting them as a better option. The problem with this thinking is that there's no evidence to suggest that one type of hormone is any better or safer than another. What little we know about the differences between the various types of estrogens and progestogens is that they all have similar effects on the body. Women who use compounded hormones need to ask the same questions about safety, risks, and benefits as for commercial hormone preparations — or for any other drug, for that matter.

The reason compounded hormones are described as "natural" or "bio-identical" is that they have the same chemical structure as the estrogen or progesterone made by a woman's body. The idea of taking something that is a chemical match to a hormone produced in your body is an appealing concept, but there's simply no scientific evidence that it's safer or better than another type of hormone.

I get frustrated when I hear compounded hormones referred to as "natural." The only natural hormones are those made inside your body. Consider what goes into producing a bio-identical version of a hormone such as estradiol, which is the dominant hormone in a woman's body before menopause. A chemist starts with a plant — usually a yam — and extracts a sterol from the cell membrane. A sterol has 17 carbon atoms. The chemist adds another carbon atom to the mix, along with some hydrogen and oxygen. Then he rearranges everything to make $C_{18}H_{24}O_2$, which is the chemical name for 17-beta estradiol. Once the ingredient is formed, additional chemicals and other compounds are added so that the hormone can be ingested and absorbed by the body.

The point is, while the estradiol itself is an exact chemical copy of the estradiol made by a woman's body, it resulted from an elaborate chemical process in a laboratory. There's nothing natural about it. It simply is not accurate to call these drugs "natural" or "identical" to a hormone made by the body. It has an identical chemical structure, but it's still a copy and not the original.

What You Get When You Buy Compounded Hormones

In addition to estradiol, two other types of estrogen are used by compounding pharmacists. One is estrone, which is the dominant estrogen found in the body after menopause. The other is estriol, a hormone produced primarily during pregnancy and present only in trace amounts at other times in a woman's life.

The most popular compounded hormones are Biest and Triest. Biest is 20 percent estradiol and 80 percent estriol. Triest is 10 percent estradiol, 10 percent estrone, and 80 percent estriol. Compounders also offer chemically identical versions of progesterone and testosterone, as well as dehydroepiandrosterone (DHEA) and pregnenolone. The latter drugs are copies of hormones produced by the adrenal glands and converted to other hormones by the body.

We have the most safety data about estradiol, which is available from commercial drug companies, as well as compounding pharmacies. The drug Estrace, for instance, contains estradiol derived from plants, just like the estradiol offered by compounders. Although most of the big studies of hormone therapy have involved Premarin or Prempro, there are several studies that have used estradiol. There's no evidence that estradiol is better or safer than other estrogens. Anecdotally, some doctors say their patients have fewer side effects while using estradiol. Other doctors say they prefer Premarin because the drug has been so well studied and because they have more experience prescribing it for their patients. For now, the FDA has advised women and their doctors to assume that every type of estrogen carries the same risks and benefits as the estrogens studied in the WHI.

We know less about the effects of estrone and estriol. In the United States, drugs containing estrone and estriol aren't commercially available and haven't been subjected to the rigorous testing requirements of the FDA. There's no reason to think that these drugs are any riskier than other hormone drugs, but there's also no evidence that they are safer or better.

Estriol is considered the weakest of the three estrogens. Proponents say that this is an advantage, because it causes fewer side effects. But it may also mean that estriol is less effective at relieving symptoms. The estrogenic potency of estriol may be 1/80 that of estradiol.[7]

In a review of the medical science on estriol, the medical journal *Menopause* found studies in which estriol seems to be effective in controlling hot flashes, insomnia, vaginal dryness, and frequent urinary tract infections associated with menopause. But estriol may not be as effective as other forms of estrogen in preventing bone loss. Some proponents say estriol helps blunt the effect of other estrogens on breast and endometrial tissue — a claim that stems from animal studies. Other research shows that estriol doesn't block other estrogens. Right now, there isn't enough evidence to back this claim.

As with other forms of estrogen, estriol stimulates endometrial tissue, which lines the uterus. Women who still have a uterus should be monitored while on estriol and likely will be prescribed a progestogen as well.[8]

The other form of estrogen used in compounded drugs is estrone. Estrone isn't found in any commercial hormone preparations in the United States. Here, it is available only through compounding pharmacies. Estrone is sold in Europe under the brand name Synapause-E_3.

An Extra Step

When most doctors prescribe hormones, they adjust the dose based on a woman's symptoms. If her symptoms get better but she's having too many side effects, the doctor might lower the dose until it's at a level at which symptoms improve and side effects are minimal. If the woman continues to suffer hot flashes, the doctor may raise the dose, checking regularly to gauge the balance between symptom relief and side effects.

Doctors who prescribe compounded hormones add an extra step to this process. They perform a saliva test, or sometimes a blood test, which measures a woman's natural hormone levels. The belief is that testing allows doctors to better determine which hormones are in short supply in a woman's body. Then they can prescribe a customized hormone mix that they say will do a better job of relieving menopausal symptoms with fewer side effects than commercial hormone preparations.

Some doctors question the reliability of saliva and other tests, saying that a woman's hormone levels vary dramatically and that hormone levels detected in saliva or blood tests haven't been proven to have anything to do with a woman's menopause symptoms. No reputable medical group supports saliva or blood testing to determine a woman's hormone levels during menopause.

Most doctors say the best approach is to judge a hormone's effectiveness by symptom relief.

Even so, many women like to know what their personal hormone levels are. If a woman goes in for regular testing, over time, she may get a sense of how the hormone levels in her body are changing. But the saliva tests and follow-up visits can get expensive. The initial doctor visit can range from $200 to $400, with follow-up visits ranging from $125 to $250 apiece and needed about every 3 months until a woman's hormones are considered "stable." Lab work from each visit can cost $100 to $400, while the hormones themselves cost $30 to $100 monthly. Many of these costs aren't covered by insurance.

According to medical groups such as the North American Menopause Society and the American College of Obstetricians and Gynecologists, there is no evidence that compounded hormones are better or safer than commercial hormone preparations. In addition, these groups have raised questions about whether compounded drugs have been adequately tested. The problem is that compounding pharmacies and the products they make exist in somewhat of a regulatory vacuum. Pharmacy practices are regulated by state pharmacy boards, while the FDA has purview over pharmaceutical companies. In the coming months, we should hear more from the FDA about its stance on compounded hormones and how consumers can best protect themselves. The American Medical Women's Association has raised concerns about the safety and purity of compounded hormones, the lack of regulation surrounding production of the hormones, and the fact that many pharmacies have made misleading marketing claims about compounded hormones.

If you're considering compounded hormones, it's important to have a long conversation with your doctor about his or her experiences with different types of hormones. Be sure to ask about a reputable pharmacy that could fill a prescription for compounded hormones. Find out how long your doctor has worked with the pharmacy, and the experience and credentials of the pharmacist who will be filling your prescription. Ask up front about the costs of testing and follow-up visits, and how much of these costs will be covered by insurance.

Compounded hormones are a reasonable option for any woman with menopausal symptoms. Doctors who prescribe compounded hormones typically work closely with their patients and schedule regular follow-up visits to make sure all is well. Just be aware that in using compounded hormones, you are assuming the same risks and benefits as for other menopause hormones outlined in this book. Overall, most doctors believe that hormones — whether they are made by commercial drug companies or compounding pharmacies — are safe and effective to treat menopausal symptoms. Be wary of a doctor or pharmacist who makes additional claims about the potential benefits of compounded hormones.

HORMONES IN BIRTH CONTROL PILLS

So what about the Pill? That's the question many women are asking as they consider the risks and benefits of menopause hormones. Birth control pills also contain forms of estrogen and progestin. Women who for years have been told that they can safely use hormones to prevent unwanted pregnancies now worry about the risks of these same hormones as they approach menopause.

Part of the reason for the confusion has to do with the way in which medicine calculates the risks and benefits of drugs. As with menopause hormones, birth control pills are associated with slightly higher risks of blood clots, strokes, and breast cancer. But women in their twenties and thirties who use birth control pills are at such low risk for these health problems to start with that even a slight increase in risk from oral contraceptive use is unlikely to make a meaningful difference. In addition, the benefits of birth control pills are obvious. Most women don't even pay attention to warnings about blood clots and stroke associated with oral contraceptives. Preventing pregnancy is just too important.

By the time a woman reaches menopause, however, the issue isn't pregnancy but overall wellness. There is such a wide range of menopause symptoms, from mild to severe, that the risk-benefit equation changes, depending on each woman's health and personal situation.

Birth control pills and menopause drugs both contain hormones that mimic the estrogen and progesterone in a woman's body. However, the actual hormones are different. For instance, Prempro, the menopause hormone studied in the WHI, contains a mixture of estrogens along with the synthetic progestin medroxyprogesterone. Other menopause hormones contain plant-derived estradiol or progesterone. On the other hand, birth control pills are made with ethinyl estradiol and synthetic progestins such as norgestimate, among others. The difference is that the hormones in birth control pills typically are more potent than the hormones in menopause drugs.

Many women assume they need high doses of hormones to cope with menopause symptoms, but menopause drugs actually have lower doses of hormones than birth control pills. That's because birth control pills have a bigger job to do — they suppress ovulation. The amount of hormone in a birth control pill is about five times higher than what is in a menopause hormone. So if you have been on the Pill and are switching to menopause hormones, you will be getting far lower quantities of estrogen and progestin. The risks are similar for both birth control pills and menopause hormones, but their impact depends on a woman's age. Package inserts included with birth control pills warn of blood clots, stroke, and heart attack. Smokers and women with high blood pressure are at highest risk. In the WHI, older women who used menopause hormones were also at higher risk for heart attack, stroke, and blood clots. The main difference is that these problems typically don't affect young women and are far more likely to show up among older women who use hormones.

In 1998, Harvard researchers reviewed nearly 400 studies looking at heart attack risk associated with oral contraceptive use. The researchers concluded that nonsmokers show little or no increase in heart attack risk from birth control pills. A woman who smokes and takes the Pill, however, has a significantly higher heart attack risk. WHI data show that women who use hormones near menopause don't have a higher heart attack risk, but their risk jumps if they start hormone therapy 10 years past menopause.

The data on breast cancer risk are a little less clear. In 1996, the medical journal *Lancet* reviewed 54 studies involving more than 150,000 women. It found that during the time a woman is on the Pill and for 10 years after stopping, she shows a modest increase in her risk of developing breast cancer. Women who began using oral contraceptives before age 20 have a slightly higher risk. In the WHI, users of combination menopause hormones (both estrogen and progestin) also had a higher risk of breast cancer after 3 years. Women who take only estrogen during menopause have no increased risk and may even receive some protection from the disease.

Taking birth control pills also lowers a

woman's risk of ovarian, colon, and uterine cancers. Menopause hormones appear to lower the risk of colon cancer, and they won't increase the risk of uterine cancer provided estrogen is paired with progestin. It's not clear how menopause hormones might influence the risk of ovarian cancer.

The bottom line is that women use high doses of estrogen and progestin to prevent pregnancy, and they use low doses of these same hormones to improve their quality of life beyond their reproductive years. The overall risks and benefits of hormones depend on a number of factors, including your age and your risk of other health problems. You and your doctor need to consider whether the potential benefits of these drugs outweigh your own personal risks.

13
HORMONE ALTERNATIVES: DRUGS, SUPPLEMENTS, AND OTHER OPTIONS

As you are making the decision about whether to use hormones during the menopausal transition, you also should consider the alternatives. Prescription drugs, herbs, vitamins, and alternative therapies like acupuncture and massage are all potential options for women who just don't want to take hormones but still need help to get through menopause. These options work for many women, but it's important for you to realize that they carry their own risks and benefits. Just because an herb or drug is not a hormone, that doesn't mean it's safer or better than a hormone. It's just different.

The fact is that we know little about most alternative treatments for menopausal symptoms. Women often turn to herbs and botanical supplements, perceiving them as more "natural" than prescription hormone preparations. While the appeal of these products is understandable, they can contain potent chemical compounds that cause druglike effects. Further, herbal and nutritional supplements aren't subjected to the same scrutiny and regulation as prescription drugs, and some products don't contain the ingredients they promise. By doing a little extra homework, women can seek out reliable products. Still, the scientific data supporting the use of supplements for menopausal symptoms are limited. This doesn't mean you shouldn't consider them, but you should be wary of exaggerated claims about their potential benefits.

Prescription drugs are another option for women who need relief from menopause symptoms but who choose not to take menopause hormones. The advantage of a prescription drug compared with an herbal supplement is that it has been subjected to rigorous testing and standards, as required by the FDA. But while drugs are a reasonable option for some women, it's important to remember that every drug carries with it a set of risks and benefits. Just because it's not a hormone doesn't mean it's safer than hormones.

Remember, too, that every woman coping with menopause can try various lifestyle changes, whether she is taking menopause hormones, other prescription drugs, supplements, or nothing at all. Lifestyle changes are a risk-free way to battle menopausal symptoms — and as a bonus, most of them will improve your overall health.

Here's a look at some non-hormone treatment options for the main health concerns of menopause: hot flashes, sleep problems, vaginal changes, and bone loss.

HOT FLASHES

Lifestyle Changes

Research shows that lifestyle changes really do make a difference in helping to curb hot flashes. Because hot flashes likely are the result of changes in the way the body regulates its temperature, keeping cool and comfortable is a good way to reduce their frequency. Dress in light clothing, use fans and air conditioners, and drink lots of cold ice water (which is good for you anyway).

Also, pay attention to what you're doing when a hot flash occurs. Some women notice that certain actions trigger a hot flash — such as consuming a hot beverage, caffeine, or alcohol or having an emotional outburst. Spicy foods, hot tubs, and even hot showers can cause trouble.

Some studies have shown that stress

management — either through therapy or activities like yoga — can lower the number of hot flashes a woman experiences each day.

Herbs/Supplements

Several herbs and supplements are touted for curbing hot flashes. Unfortunately, the data are limited, though there is some evidence that some alternative remedies may make a modest difference. If you remain wary of menopause hormones or certain prescription drugs, it may make sense for you to try an herb or supplement along with lifestyle changes.

If you go this route, take some time to check out the various supplements sold in drugstores and health food stores. As mentioned earlier, herbs and supplements aren't subjected to the same strict regulations as prescription drugs. There have been numerous reports of adulterated products or products containing only trace amounts of the ingredients identified on the label.

One excellent Web site for checking out various supplement brands is www.consumerlab.com, an independent firm that tests supplements to determine if they contain the promised ingredients. Detailed reports are available for a fee. Products that pass

ConsumerLab's testing may carry the CL seal on their labels. The nonprofit U.S. Pharmacopeia offers its USP seal to products that pass its testing program. Be sure to look for bottles that contain the USP or CL safety seals.

While supplement manufacturers are required to adhere to the government's food-processing standards, some voluntarily adhere to the higher manufacturing standards imposed on drugs. The product labels may reflect that. The bottom line: If you choose an herbal or nutritional supplement, do your homework to make sure you're getting a quality product. Among the supplements you might want to consider:

Black cohosh. Black cohosh appears to be one of the most promising nonprescription treatments for hot flashes. Compared with other non-hormonal treatments, black cohosh has been relatively well researched, although the data so far are mixed. One study showed that black cohosh reduced hot flashes by 84 percent.[1] In another, the herb worked just as well as estrogen in reducing hot flashes.[2] Still others have found black cohosh to have little if any benefit.

It's not clear how black cohosh might work. It may act like an estrogen in the body, or it may be more like a selective estrogen receptor modulator, or SERM. A SERM is a drug that acts like estrogen on some tissues but blocks the effects of estrogen on other tissues. Black cohosh may also decrease luteinizing hormone, a hormone secreted by the pituitary gland that may play a role in hot flashes.

There are no obvious adverse effects from black cohosh. As with other supplements, long-term risks and benefits aren't known.

Soy. Soy contains large quantities of isoflavones, plant compounds that are similar to estrogens. In the body, they compete with estrogen for the same receptors and have estrogen-like effects. But they don't appear to be nearly as effective as estrogens in curbing hot flashes. One small study of 39 women showed a 20 percent improvement in hot flashes.[3] Another study found that women who used soy had just as many hot flashes, but they were less severe than in women who didn't use soy.[4] In a study of 75 women, soy users experienced a 61 percent drop in hot flashes compared with a 21 percent decline among placebo users.[5] Several other studies have not found any benefit from soy use.[6]

Although the data are mixed, it does appear that soy isoflavones may help some women cope with hot flashes. It's important to remember that soy acts like an estrogen, albeit a mild one, in the body. In one study that looked at the impact of soy isoflavones on the uterus, soy users didn't experience any more changes in the uterine lining than non-soy users.[7] However, the effects of long-term use aren't known.

Red clover. Despite anecdotal reports that red clover helps with hot flashes, there's little evidence to support this. One study of just 30 women did show that red clover users had 44 percent fewer hot flashes than placebo users.[8] However, two small studies did not show any benefit from red clover.[9] None of the studies reported any adverse effects from the herb, but long-term risks and benefits aren't known.

Other agents. Dong quai, vitamin E, evening primrose oil, ginseng, melatonin, and wild yam are all talked about as potentially effective against hot flashes. Unfortunately, there's no solid scientific evidence to back up such claims.

Prescription Drugs

Antidepressants. Perhaps the biggest change in menopause treatment in the past few years has been the widespread prescribing of antidepressants to treat hot flashes. The use of antidepressants for hot flashes is a little disconcerting given that historically, menopausal women were treated as hysterical when they complained about the physical and mental changes triggered by menopause. Though antidepressants have not been approved by the FDA as a hot-flash remedy, doctors now prescribe them "off label" for this purpose.

Antidepressants act by increasing levels of a brain chemical called serotonin. While the drugs are effective against depression, nobody really knows how or why altering a woman's brain chemistry might work to relieve hot flashes. Since we do know that hot flashes originate in the brain, it may be that adjusting a woman's serotonin levels affects the part of her brain that controls body temperature. Another theory is that serotonin influences levels of a woman's natural estrogen.

Researchers first discovered the link between antidepressants and hot flashes after studying women with breast cancer who were undergoing anti-estrogen therapy, which can trigger hot flashes. The women who were also taking the antidepressant Effexor seemed to have fewer hot flashes than women who weren't taking the antidepressant.

Unfortunately, most of what we know

about antidepressants and hot flashes comes from two studies involving a total of 386 women who took the drugs for 6 weeks or less. According to a *Journal of the American Medical Association (JAMA)* review and analysis of studies of antidepressants as a treatment for hot flashes, antidepressants work only about one-third as well as hormones in reducing hot flashes.[10]

The two antidepressants that show the most promise are Paxil and Effexor. In the best Paxil trial, women taking the antidepressant experienced one less hot flash a day than women taking a placebo. The Effexor trial looked at three different doses of the drug. At the lowest dose, Effexor reduced hot flashes by just 37 percent, compared to 27 percent for the placebo. At 75 and 150 milligrams, the drug reduced hot flashes by about 60 percent. But there was a downside. The women who were taking the two largest doses also experienced the most side effects, including loss of appetite, dry mouth, nausea, and constipation.[11]

One side effect of antidpressants that may be particularly disconcerting to menopausal women is loss of libido. At a time in a woman's life when fluctuating hormone levels already may be playing havoc with her sex drive, it's important to be aware of this potential side effect. Wyeth is studying a new antidepressant called Pristiq for the treatment of hot flashes. The company says that in its early studies, the incidence of diminished libido wasn't any different with Pristiq than with placebo.

Beyond loss of sexual interest, antidepressants have been shown to interfere with basic emotions. Rutgers University anthropologist Helen Fisher, PhD, has conducted brain-scan studies in which antidepressants appear to blunt important emotions related to love, romance, and long-term attachment. They may do this by interfering with dopamine, a brain chemical connected with emotions and the sense of pleasure.

Doctors also have raised questions about the effect of antidepressants in women with normal brain chemistry who aren't depressed. It is known that taking antidepressants results in certain changes in brain receptors. That's why people who try to stop the medications sometimes develop severe withdrawal symptoms until the brain receptors return to normal.

There's no reason to think that antidepressants aren't safe; they've been used for years by millions of patients. But many questions remain about their long-term risks and benefits as a treatment for hot flashes.

Other drugs. Two other prescription drugs, the blood pressure medicine clonidine and the antiseizure medicine gabapentin (Neurontin), may help reduce hot flashes.

Sleep Problems

Many women develop sleep problems during menopause. It's no wonder. The hormonal chaos and the personal and professional issues that are common at midlife would be enough to keep any woman up at night. Hot flashes — called night sweats when they happen at night — can significantly interfere with sleep. Estrogen clearly helps reduce hot flashes, and it's also known to improve the quality of sleep in postmenopausal women. A side effect of progesterone is sleepiness, so taking it at night can help improve sleep. But if you've decided against hormone therapy, you still have other options for getting a better night's sleep.

Lifestyle Changes

Pretty much everyone could benefit from better sleep hygiene. That means improving your habits in the evening as you prepare for bedtime. It may not solve 100 percent of the sleep problems sometimes associated with menopause, but it's a good start. Here are some common suggestions for improving sleep:

Establish a regular bedtime and wake-up time. Keep to a schedule. Staying up late and sleeping in on weekends throws off your brain circuitry and can interfere with sleep.

Resist naps. Taking a quick catnap during the day might help reinvigorate you, but it also may be interfering with your sleep schedule and your ability to fall asleep at night, creating a vicious cycle of poor sleep and midday sleepiness.

Skip the late-night cocktail. Drinking alcohol may make you sleepy at first, but after a few hours, it can have a stimulant effect. Try to avoid alcohol for 4 to 6 hours before bedtime.

Eliminate caffeine. Caffeine is great for keeping us alert during the day. Often, though, it stays with us longer than we want it to. A morning cup of coffee and a diet cola in the afternoon may ruin your bedtime. If you can't give it up entirely, try to limit caffeine intake to the early part of the day, avoiding it for at least 6 hours before bedtime. Remember that chocolate has caffeine, too.

Watch what and when you eat. Avoiding big meals, spicy foods, and late-night eating is a good way to improve your sleep. It's also smart to steer clear of starchy or sugary foods in the evening, because they can cause a glucose surge that keeps you up at night.

Treat heartburn. Heartburn often interferes with sleep. If you have regular heartburn, talk to your doctor about treatment. Several over-the-counter drugs as well as some prescription drugs are highly effective in relieving heartburn. Chronic heartburn sufferers also should learn to sleep on their left side, which can help alleviate symptoms.

Exercise, but not at bedtime. Regular physical activity improves sleep quality, but working out within a few hours of bedtime can leave you energized and alert just when you don't want to be.

Don't watch TV in bed. Most of us do it, but if you're having trouble with sleep, take the television out of the bedroom. For many people, television is just too stimulating and interesting, and it keeps them from falling asleep.

Check your sleep environment. Make sure you have a comfy mattress and bedding. Turn off the lights, and make sure your shades are blocking out light.

Herbs/Supplements

A number of herbal remedies are popular treatments for insomnia and sleep problems. Valerian, passionflower, St. John's wort, black cohosh, hops, skullcap, and chamomile have all been touted as helpful for this purpose. As is often the case with herbal remedies, there aren't enough well-designed studies to prove the herbs' sleep-inducing effects. Many women swear by herbal teas as helpful in calming nerves and bringing on sleep.

Prescription Drugs

A number of prescription drugs are useful for treating sleep problems, but you need to talk with your doctor about how and when best to use them. One concern about treating the sleep problems associated with menopause is that the menopausal transition can last for 2 to 3 years, if not longer. Most doctors prefer to prescribe pharmaceutical sleep aids as short-term treatments for sleep problems but discourage long-term use. Beyond the fact that many of these drugs stop working with long-term use, doctors also worry about patients becoming dependent on the drugs.

Some of the newer sleep aids address some of these worries. Compared with old-line sleep therapies, these drugs carry fewer side effects, are less likely to cause grogginess the next day, are less likely to be abused or cause dependence, and are less likely to lose effectiveness over time. As a result, some of the newer sleep aids, such as Ambien and Lunesta, may be an option for menopausal women dealing with sleep problems.

In one 4-week Harvard study, the drug Ambien was found to be effective for treating sleep problems in perimenopausal and postmenopausal women.[12] It was a short study, but it did show that non-hormone treatments can help improve sleep quality in women coping with menopausal symptoms. The hormone melatonin also may be prescribed for postmenopausal sleep problems.

Vaginal Dryness/Atrophy
Lifestyle Changes
Since vaginal aging is an inevitable part of getting older, every woman should think about lifestyle and self-care issues associated with vaginal health, whether or not she chooses to use menopause hormones. Sexual exercise is one of the best things you can do for your vagina as you get older. Having regular sex quite literally keeps your

vagina in shape. Women who have sex more often are less likely to report problems with vaginal dryness and itching. In one study of about 50 women between ages 50 and 65, the women who had intercourse at least three times a month experienced significantly less urogenital atrophy than women who were sexually inactive.[13]

If regular sex with a partner isn't an option, regular use of a vibrator or dildo is recommended. Avoid douches, soaps, bubble baths, and lotions that irritate the vaginal area. And nothing gets in the way of a relaxed sex life more than stress. Consider counseling, regular outings with friends, and exercise as ways to relieve the stress burden of midlife.

Lubricants and Moisturizers

Studies have found that lubricants and moisturizers are useful in treating vaginal dryness. Unlike menopause hormones, however, they are a short-term solution.

Lubricants such as Astroglide and K-Y Jelly need to be used regularly and reapplied before sex to be effective. Be sure to read product labels because certain types of petroleum-based lubricants can interact with latex and reduce the strength of condoms.

Vaginal moisturizers, including the brand Replens, can have a longer-term effect, requiring application only two or three times a week. In addition, they don't need to be reapplied before sex. Notably, one study compared Replens applied three times a week with vaginal estrogen cream used daily. Replens worked just as well as the estrogen to relieve symptoms.[14]

Herbal Products

A number of herbal products are touted as solutions to vaginal dryness. Among them are agrimony, black cohosh, ginseng, motherwort, chaste tree, dong quai, witch hazel, phytoestrogens, and wild yam creams. As is often the case with herbal remedies, there is little or no evidence to support the therapeutic claims for these products.[15]

BONE HEALTH

Lifestyle Changes

The best thing you can do for your bones is to stay physically active, whether or not you are taking estrogen after menopause. Weight-bearing exercise does the most to protect your bone health, so focus on activities like walking, running, and aerobics that keep you moving on your feet. Exercise not only keeps bones strong, it also improves balance, flexibility, and agility — meaning that people who work out simply are more sure on their feet and less likely to fall and hurt themselves. An elderly person with severe osteoporosis who never falls is better off than an elderly person with healthy bones who regularly takes a spill.

Although there are many health reasons to stop smoking, bone health is a big one. Cigarette smoking may impair calcium absorption and reduce natural estrogen levels. Studies show that women smokers lose bone more rapidly, have lower bone mass, and reach menopause as much as 2 years sooner than nonsmokers.[16]

Heavy alcohol consumption is known to increase the risk of falls and hip fracture. One study found that as few as two drinks a day increases the risk of fracture.[17]

Herbs/Supplements

Calcium/vitamin D. Menopause hormones weren't the only subject of the Women's Health Initiative (WHI). It also looked at whether calcium and vitamin D are effective treatments for bone health. The interpretation of the calcium data from the WHI study and the accompanying publicity was confusing to women. It left many with the impression that calcium doesn't improve bone health. The fact is that calcium works — and works quite well — to protect your bones, but only if you take it regularly.

The WHI tracked calcium use in 36,000 women. The overall finding was that calcium didn't make much of a difference to their bone health, a result that sparked widespread news stories questioning whether postmenopausal women should adhere to federal guidelines recommending 1,200 milligrams of calcium a day. But WHI researchers now say that the data have been largely misinterpreted by the public. The overall finding isn't really a reliable indicator of calcium's effects. For one thing, the results were skewed by the fact that the study included women under age 60, who generally aren't at risk for fractures. In addition, many women in the placebo group were taking calcium supplements on the side. By the end of the study, only 59 percent of the women in both the placebo and the control groups were consistently taking the study pills.

All these problems clouded the data, making the trends that emerged in certain groups even more remarkable. Women over age 60 in the calcium group were 21 percent less likely to suffer a hip fracture than women in the placebo group. The benefits were even higher among just the women who took their pills regularly. Across all age groups, these women had a 29 percent lower risk of hip fracture. And among all age groups and compliance levels, women who weren't taking calcium supplements before the study reduced their risk of hip fracture by 30 percent once they began supplementation. A hip fracture is a serious health concern that almost always requires surgery and can lead to permanent disability and even death.

The biggest concern right now is that many women have begun to doubt the benefits of calcium at a time when important safety questions are being raised about other bone treatments. In the WHI hormone studies, menopause hormones lowered the risk of hip fracture by 33 percent among users of estrogen and progestin and by 35 percent among women taking estrogen alone. Among hormone users who also took calcium, the risk of fracture dropped by 60 percent.

Calcium is a relatively low-risk treatment. The WHI found that the most significant negative effect of daily calcium supplementation is a 17 percent increase in the risk of kidney stones. An Australian study found constipation to be the only side effect of calcium use.

Isoflavones. As mentioned earlier, isoflavones are estrogen-like compounds found in soybeans and soy products, as well as in red clover. They are widely touted as useful nondrug treatments for various menopause symptoms because they appear to have mild estrogen-like effects. There are some limited data to suggest that isoflavones are good for bones. But most studies, including a recent review by the North American Menopause Society, don't support their use for boosting bone health.

Other herbs. A number of other herbal remedies are touted as beneficial for bones, including black cohosh, dong quai, fennel, anise, motherwort, wild yam root, and sarsaparilla. As with other claims made about herbal products, these simply aren't backed by science.

Prescription Drugs

There are several prescription drugs besides estrogen that have been documented to improve bone health. Just like estrogen, they carry a range of risks and benefits. Before you decide to use a prescription bone therapy, you should ask a lot of questions about why your doctor thinks you need it. As we discussed earlier in this book, it's perfectly normal to have declining bone density as you age. Just because your bone health is changing, that doesn't necessarily mean you need drug therapy for it. The real question is whether other risk factors, besides a bone-density score, have prompted your doctor to suggest a prescription bone drug.

One of the biggest problems with prescription bone drugs is that women stop taking them. In various studies lasting 6 months to a year, as many as 19 to 75 percent of women discontinued treatment. This may be because some bone therapies are inconvenient, because the side effects can be unpleasant, or simply because declining bone health doesn't cause any obvious symptoms.

Bisphosphonates. If your doctor is considering a bone drug, a likely first choice is a bisphosphonate. This class of drugs is sold under various brand names, including Fosamax, Actonel, and Boniva. The drugs work by reducing bone resorption, helping to maintain and rebuild bones.

Bisphosphonates clearly help to increase bone mineral density at the spine and hip, and studies have shown that they also reduce the risk of vertebral and hip fractures.[18] Most of the available data on bisphosphonates comes from daily pills, though some weekly and monthly therapies have recently been introduced. These appear to do just as good a job of maintaining and improving bone density as the daily regimens.

Side effects of bisphosphonates can include esophageal problems, heartburn, and ulcers. In rare cases, a flulike illness might result. There is a theoretical concern about the long-term risks of bisphosphonate use. Because these drugs work to suppress bone turnover, questions have emerged about whether long-term use will make bones more brittle. There are some anecdotal cases of this, but not enough to conclude whether it's a meaningful risk.

Another potential side effect of bisphosphonates is osteonecrosis of the jaw, in which a patient's jawbone rots and dies. While the complication sounds scary, women who are using bisphosphonates shouldn't panic. Merck, the maker of Fosamax, notes that in 10 years of clinical trials involving more than 17,000 patients, there have been no reports of osteonecrosis of the jaw.

While the disease remains rare, numerous cases that have shown up in the medical literature appear to be linked with bisphosphonate use. The majority of people suffering from osteonecrosis of the jaw are cancer patients taking a potent intravenous form of the drug to stop cancer cells from dissolving bone. A small number of cases have also been reported among noncancer patients using oral bisphosphonates. Doctors say these patients typically have used the drugs for 7 to 8 years.

It's simply not clear who is at risk for osteonecrosis of the jaw. Some doctors advise patients taking drugs such as Fosamax to avoid major dental or oral surgery if they can. Such surgery may be the trigger of problems, because the jawbone is slow to heal, and complications can develop.

Selective estrogen receptor modulators (SERMS). As mentioned earlier, a SERM is a drug that acts like estrogen on some tissues but blocks the effect of estrogen on other tissues. The SERM raloxifene, sold under the brand name Evista, has been shown to boost bone density and slow bone turnover. An important study called MORE (for Multiple Outcomes of Raloxifene Evaluation) found that the overall incidence of fracture dropped by 72 percent after 4 years of treatment with raloxifene. The drug, which is in the same class as tamoxifen, also appeared to lower the risk of breast cancer. While there was a significant increase in health problems related to blood clots, that didn't appear to alter risk of heart attack or stroke.

The big downside of raloxifene is that it may increase hot flashes. Also, bone loss continues once treatment stops.

Calcitonin. Calcitonin, which includes the brands Miacalcin, Calcimar, and Fortical, is a naturally occurring hormone that affects calcium regulation and bone metabolism. Calcitonin slows bone loss and increases spinal bone density. It also reduces the risk of spinal fractures, though it has not been shown to decrease the risk of nonspine fractures.

Calcitonin is available only as an injection or a nasal spray. Side effects of injectable calcitonin may include flushing of the face and hands, nausea, skin rash, and increased urinary frequency. Side effects of nasal calcitonin are less common but may include nasal irritation, back pain, bloody nose, and headaches.

Parathyroid hormone (PTH). In cases of severe osteoporosis and high fracture risk, doctors may suggest PTH, sold under the brand name Forteo. Doctors also prescribe Forteo for patients who can't tolerate other osteoporosis drugs. It is different from other drugs in that it stimulates new bone formation by increasing the number and activity of bone-forming cells. By comparison, drugs like Fosamax are antiresorptives, which slow the activity of bone-removing cells. Both types of drugs improve bone density, although Forteo likely will do it faster.

Forteo isn't recommended for everyone because the drug carries some significant risks. In rat studies, it was linked with a type of bone cancer. Although the risk hasn't been seen in humans, right now, Forteo can be used for only 24 months. In addition, the drug carries a so-called black box warning, which the FDA requires to alert patients to potentially serious health risks.

Forteo is administered as a daily injection. It is expensive, costing about $600 a month.

14
THE HORMONE DECISION

Now that you understand the science behind menopause hormones, it's time for you to make your own personal hormone decision. Choosing whether or not to use menopause hormones is a different enterprise today than it was even 10 years ago. Chances are that your mother, your aunts, and your older women friends all believed not only that hormones helped hot flashes but also that every woman, regardless of her symptoms, should stay on hormones for the rest of her life. In recent years, the pendulum swung to the other extreme, as many women became convinced that hormones caused heart attacks and breast cancer and that no woman, no matter how much she was suffering from hot flashes and other menopausal symptoms, should ever use hormones.

Today, the pendulum has swung again — but this time it is hovering somewhere in the middle of those two extremes. We know that hormones are not a fountain of youth, nor are they as risky as they have been portrayed. They are clearly the most effective option for relieving hot flashes caused by menopause, and they help preserve bone and vaginal health. But menopause hormones also carry some slight risks that require thoughtful consideration. For example, they definitely increase the risk of blood clots. And while breast cancer is probably not a worry for women who take only estrogen, women who take a combination of estrogen and progestin do have to think about a possible increase in risk after several years of use.

We know that starting hormone therapy has no benefit for older women who are long past menopause and that according to all the evidence, older women who start taking hormones long past menopause face a higher risk of heart attack and stroke. But we don't yet fully understand the impact of hormone therapy on the heart attack risk, stroke risk, and brain health of young women who are just starting the menopausal transition. Many in the medical community remain convinced that when the Women's Health Initiative (WHI) data are broken down, they actually show that menopause hormones aren't risky to women who are still close to menopause and that they could offer extra heart protection. Future research will help shed light on all these issues.

But women who are coping with menopause symptoms right now don't have years to wait for answers. They must rely on the information that is available today. The good news is, there is a tremendous amount of data to help women with their hormone decision.

While the WHI has generated headlines that have scared women away from menopause hormones, I have long believed that the WHI has provided some of the most reassuring data to date about the benefits and risks of hormone therapy. The problem is not the study or the results but how they have been interpreted. Harvard gynecologist Alan M. Altman, MD, a firm believer in the benefits of hormone therapy, compares the data from the WHI with the data found on a driver's license. The basic facts are all there — name, age, height, sex, and even eye color. You wouldn't think there's much room for disagreement in reading the data from a driver's license. But show a woman's license to her school-age child, and the child will conclude that his mother got an "F" in sex. "The data can be right there in front of you," Dr. Altman says. "It's how you interpret the data that matters."

And so, now it is up to you and your doctor to consider all the WHI data and other research on menopause hormones as you make your own personal hormone decision. Hormone therapy is not a one-size-fits-all proposition. Hormones are not good for all women, nor are they bad for all women. The question is whether they are right or wrong for you.

How to Make the Hormone Decision

Ever since the release of the WHI results, doctors around the country have been struggling to advise women on hormone therapy. Most experts now believe that the most important lesson of the WHI may be to "individualize" the hormone decision to each woman. But what exactly does that mean?

Several medical groups have tried to come up with guidelines for doctors and their patients. Many doctors think that because the WHI involved primarily older women, the overall results shouldn't be a factor in the hormone decision of a younger woman who's coping with menopause symptoms. However, public awareness of the risks and benefits of menopause hormones is so heavily influenced by the WHI that it probably makes most sense to consider the data from the WHI along with all the other evidence about hormone therapy.

That's what researchers did for a *British Medical Journal (BMJ)* article in which they attempted to create a clinical decision analysis to advise doctors on how best to prescribe menopause hormones.[1] They didn't argue against the WHI, or make the point that it applies only to older women, or debate whether the breast cancer and heart data are misleading. They just accepted the WHI data as valid and used the research as a starting point to advise doctors and women about hormones. As part of their analysis, they also used quality-of-life data from other studies in an attempt to balance the risks identified in the WHI against the benefits of symptom relief — an issue that the WHI wasn't designed to address.

The results are surprising. Accepting the worst-case scenario about the risks of menopause hormones, the *BMJ* analysis still concluded that *the benefits of hormones to women with menopause symptoms outweigh the risks during 5 years of use.* The same article concluded that women with no symptoms face more risks than benefits if they choose to use menopause hormones.

The results of the *BMJ* study offer a reassuring starting point for evaluating the pros and cons of hormone use for an individual woman. But given that every hormone decision should be based on a woman's own risks, symptoms, concerns, and expectations, the *BMJ* report also shouldn't be viewed as the final word on hormone therapy.

TELLING YOUR HEALTH STORY

Whether menopause hormones are right for you depends on your personal and family health history, your current symptoms, and your own beliefs about taking medication on a regular basis. Here are some first steps and questions that will help you weigh the risks and benefits of hormone therapy.

Assess your symptoms. Write down what menopause symptoms you are experiencing right now. Do you find yourself constantly thinking about menopause? Are your symptoms disrupting your home and work life? Have you noticed changes in your mood and sleep patterns, and what kind of effect are those changes having on your life? Have you found that your memory is slipping, or your thinking sometimes seems fuzzy? Do you feel as though your symptoms are worse than those of other women you know, about average, or fairly mild? Talking to other women about their experiences during menopause will help give you perspective, though in the end, it's about how you feel and how manageable or severe you believe your symptoms are.

If you have hot flashes, think about how many you have and how long they last. Typically, a woman is considered to have severe menopause symptoms if she has seven or more hot flashes a day. But that really depends on the woman and what she's doing at the time of the hot flash. A busy executive would probably find even two hot flashes a day to be unacceptable if they interfere with her ability to perform effectively. On the other hand, a woman who works in a more casual atmosphere or is surrounded by female colleagues might find coping with hot flashes to be easier in such a relaxed and supportive environment. A woman who is retired or has a lot of leisure time might find herself laughing off her regular bouts of hot flashes or better able to cool down with cold water or air-conditioning in the privacy of her home. But if that woman is a caregiver to a relative or children, hot flashes might still be inconvenient, if not disruptive.

There are so many different scenarios, it's impossible to describe them all. What matters is how you are feeling. Take your own personal symptom assessment and discuss it with your doctor. Tracking which symptoms you're experiencing, how they're affecting your life, and whether they are mild, moderate, or severe will help your doctor better advise you.

Here's a list of common menopausal symptoms for which hormone therapy can offer relief. Put a check mark next to the symptoms you're experiencing and note how often they occur.

Hot flashes	_____	_____
Night sweats	_____	_____
Sleep problems	_____	_____
Mood changes	_____	_____
Depression	_____	_____
Fuzzy thinking	_____	_____
Memory problems	_____	_____
Body aches	_____	_____
Irregular bleeding	_____	_____
Urinary tract infections	_____	_____
Vaginal dryness	_____	_____
Vaginal itching/discomfort	_____	_____
Painful sex	_____	_____
Low sex drive	_____	_____

Consider the side effects. Here are some common side effects of menopause hormones. Although they typically affect only a small percentage of women, you should still ask yourself whether they seem manageable or unacceptable to you.

Common Side Effects
Breast tenderness
Fluid retention
Pelvic cramping
Breakthrough bleeding

Migraines (though some women actually experience migraine relief)
Bloating
Stomach upset/nausea
Hair loss

Less Common but Serious Side Effects
Breast lumps
Changes in vaginal bleeding
Dizziness
Fainting
Vision changes
Chest pain
Shortness of breath
Leg pain
Vomiting

Assess your health. Are you a healthy person? Are you overweight? Do you exercise regularly? If you are healthy, your overall risk for the types of health problems identified in the WHI (heart attack, stroke, breast cancer) is most likely low. Even if you assume the worst-case scenario about the risks associated with hormone use, you may not have much to worry about. Your starting point for risk is low, so your overall risk will remain low, even with an added bump from hormone use.

On the other hand, if you smoke, don't

exercise, and are overweight, your risk of health problems already is on the rise, even without menopause hormones. For a body in a compromised state, even a modest increase in risk from hormone therapy may not be a good idea. Use this time in your life to reassess your health priorities and put yourself on the course to better health.

Consider your personal and family health history. Do you have a history of blood clots? Have you suffered a stroke or heart attack? Have you had breast cancer, or are you at high risk for it? Did your mother suffer any broken bones or fractures? Has your doctor told you that you are at risk for poor bone health as you get older? Use the checklist below to track your and your family's health history, as this information is vital to your hormone decision.

The most relevant family history involves your immediate family — parents or siblings who have had these health problems. But grandparents, uncles, and aunts on both sides of your family matter, too. Be sure to note the age at which a family member is diagnosed with a particular health problem. An illness that occurs in someone who's relatively young (typically before age 60) is considered significant to your health. But an illness that occurs in a family member who's in his or her seventies or eighties is usually considered normal aging and not as relevant to your personal health.

	Personal History	Family History
Heart disease		
Stroke		
Breast cancer		
Blood clots		
Osteoporosis		
Bone fractures		
Uterine cancer		
Colon cancer		
Ovarian cancer		
Gallbladder disease		

DIFFERENT WOMEN, DIFFERENT ANSWERS

Now that you've got a sense of your own health story, including your menopause symptoms and your family and personal health history, it's time to decide what health issues matter most to you. It may be that osteoporosis is a huge concern in your life. If that's the case, you likely will come up with a different hormone decision than the woman who has a strong family history and high personal risk of breast cancer. A woman who's suffering from vaginal pain due to aging is more likely to consider vaginal hormone therapy than a woman who is debilitated by daily hot flashes.

The various potential health issues faced by menopausal women result in, quite literally, hundreds of different health scenarios. Recognizing the various permutations that could influence a woman's personal hormone decision, the North American Menopause Society (NAMS) convened a panel of experts to try to come up with advice for doctors and women about when to consider menopause hormones and when to rule them out. They focused on the most serious health issues associated with hormone therapy and whether it was appropriate, inappropriate, or uncertain to use menopause hormones in low- or standard-dose pills or as patches. The American College of Obstetricians and Gynecologists (ACOG) took a similar approach, convening a task force to help advise doctors and women about hormone therapy.

Both groups have come up with general guidelines to help women and their doctors make individualized hormone decisions. Here's what they had to say about the biggest risks and benefits of menopause hormones.

Hot Flashes and Night Sweats

The ACOG task force concluded that menopause hormones are the most effective treatment, reducing hot flashes by up to 90 percent. They also recommend that women adopt lifestyle changes such as wearing lightweight clothing, maintaining cool room temperatures, and avoiding spicy foods, caffeine, and alcohol.

If you are a generally healthy person, and your hot flashes are severe or disruptive to your life, hormones are likely a good option for you. However, if you have a family history of cardiovascular disease, breast cancer, or blood clots, then you have other issues to consider before making the hormone decision.

The ACOG panel advises women to use the lowest effective dose for the shortest possible time and to reevaluate hormone therapy every year. The NAMS panel says that an annual reevaluation isn't enough and that women should regularly consider lowering the hormone dose or stopping treatment altogether. The ACOG panel notes that about 10 percent of menopausal women will continue to have vasomotor symptoms beyond the average 4 years it takes such symptoms to resolve. "It is inappropriate to withhold HT [hormone therapy] from persistently symptomatic women who prefer to continue HT or who do not derive relief from currently available alternatives," according to the ACOG report.

Blood Clots

In deep vein thrombosis, a relatively uncommon condition, blood clots form in the large blood vessels of the legs. Small clots generally don't cause any trouble, but large clots can block bloodflow and cause pain. In rare cases, a clot breaks loose and travels up the leg to the lungs, which can be fatal.

Blood clots can be caused by changes in blood circulation, which can slow when you are seated for long periods of time without moving, such as during a long plane or car trip. The risk of blood clots increases after surgery or a hip fracture or when you have another serious illness such as a heart attack or stroke. If you have had a blood clot in the past, you may be at higher risk for having one again. Often, a woman known to be at high risk for blood clots will be on drug or aspirin treatment to help keep a new clot from forming. Although it's not common, some people have a family tendency toward blood clots.

In the WHI, the risk of blood clots was clearly higher for women taking menopause hormones than for those who didn't use hormones. However, the overall risk remained low. Among estrogen and progestin users, 34 of 10,000 women developed blood clots, compared with just 16 of 10,000 who were taking placebo. Among estrogen-only users, 21 of 10,000 developed clots, compared with 15 of 10,000 non-estrogen users.

Women who have a history of blood clots or who are at risk for them must carefully weigh this information if they are considering menopause hormones for symptom relief. The ACOG panel says doctors need to advise women about the two-fold increase in blood clot risk that occurs with hormone use. For the average woman, the risk remains low. However, if you've already had blood clots, or you are known to be at higher risk, the added risk of hormone therapy may not be acceptable.

For otherwise healthy women who have undergone a hysterectomy and are at increased blood clot risk, the NAMS panel concluded that it's appropriate to prescribe an estrogen patch to relieve menopausal symptoms. Blood clot risk is believed to be lower with patch treatment than with oral estrogens. For women who still have a uterus (meaning they need both estrogen and progestin) and are at increased blood clot risk, the answer isn't as clear. The NAMS panel says it's uncertain whether a woman at a higher risk for blood clots can safely use low-dose hormones in pill or patch form. The ACOG panel says all women should be counseled about blood clot risk.

Every woman who uses menopause hormones should take precautions to prevent blood clots. Keep your legs moving. If you are in bed for a long time because of an illness, be sure to do leg and foot exercises several times a day. On a long flight or car trip, take breaks and walk around as often as possible. These are things all women should be doing anyway, whether or not they choose hormone therapy.

Heart Attack

The WHI and other important studies have shown that a woman with a history of heart attack or heart disease should not take menopause hormones. The impact of hormone therapy on the heart health of women who start using it close to menopause is not yet fully understood. Many in the medical community remain convinced that when the WHI data are broken down, they actually show that hormones aren't risky to women who are still close to menopause and may actually be beneficial to the heart. This theory is supported by a voluminous amount of data from animal and observational research, including the WHI's own observational study, which suggests that women reap heart benefits from taking hormones at the onset of menopause.

Still, there are many unanswered questions about the timing of hormone use in terms of when hormones are helpful and when they cause harm. In the view of most experts, the WHI has raised enough questions that women shouldn't take hormones in the hope of preventing heart disease or helping their hearts. However, the WHI data should be reassuring to the typical woman who's considering menopause hormones. The NAMS panel notes that women at higher risk for heart disease should consider patch hormone therapy rather than oral hormones.

To learn more about your personal risk of heart disease, take the health quiz at www.yourdiseaserisk.com.

Stroke

Just as with blood clots, menopause hormones appear to increase the risk of stroke. However, since the typical menopausal woman is younger than age 55, her overall risk of stroke remains low. So any additional risk caused by hormone therapy is unlikely to dramatically change a woman's absolute risk of stroke.

The ACOG panel recommends that healthy women be counseled regarding the small but real increase in stroke risk associated with hormone use. The NAMS panel says that women known to be at higher stroke risk should not use menopause hormones.

Women can help protect themselves against stroke by not smoking; managing blood pressure, cholesterol, and diabetes; staying active; eating a healthful diet; and maintaining a healthful weight.

To learn more about your personal stroke risk, take the quiz at www.yourdiseaserisk .com.

Breast Cancer

For many women, the breast cancer question will be the most complicated component of their personal hormone decision. For women at average breast cancer risk, here's what to think about.

If you are a woman who has undergone a hysterectomy and will take only estrogen: Data from both the WHI and the Nurses' Health Study paint the clearest picture yet of how long women who've had a hysterectomy can use estrogen therapy. Overall, there's no statistically significant increase in breast cancer risk for up to 20 years of estrogen use. After 20 years, breast cancer risk goes up slightly for estrogen users, although for breast cancers that are responsive to both estrogen and progestin, risk rose at the 15-year mark. Fifteen to 20 years is far longer than most women would ever consider using menopause hormones.

The Nurses' Health Study suggested that estrogen may lower breast cancer risk during the first 10 years of use, while according to the WHI, an average of 7 years of estrogen use could lower breast cancer risk. The bottom line for women who take only estrogen is that we have strong data to show that the hormone doesn't increase breast cancer risk for the first 7 to 10 years and may be safe for up to 15 to 20 years.

If you are a woman with a uterus and will take estrogen and progestin: Most of the scientific data suggest that women who take both estrogen and progestin do have a slightly higher risk of breast cancer than women who don't take hormones. However, the overall risk to an individual woman is still small. The ACOG panel notes that according to the overall WHI data, a woman's risk of developing breast cancer while using combination hormone therapy was *less than one-tenth of 1 percent a year.* The risk may be even lower for the typical woman considering menopause hormones.

The most important relevant data from the WHI looked at breast cancer risk among women who had never used menopause hormones before. These women most closely resemble the typical woman seeking relief from menopausal symptoms, because their breasts hadn't been exposed to hormone therapy. Women in the WHI who had never used menopause hormones but started taking them for the study were 9 percent more likely to be diagnosed with breast cancer than women who never took hormones at all. A 9 percent increase in risk is relatively small and far less scary than many of the headlines about hormone therapy and breast cancer risk would have you believe. Consider this: A 50-year-old woman may have a 2 percent chance of being diagnosed with breast cancer in the next 5 years. If her risk increases by 9 percent once she begins hormone therapy, her overall breast cancer risk remains just 2.2 percent.

To put this in perspective, talk with your doctor about your personal breast cancer risk before using hormones. There are two Web sites that can also help you gauge your breast cancer risk. One of them, www.cancer.gov/bcrisktool/, asks you to input some basic information about your health. From this information, it will calculate your baseline breast cancer risk before using menopause hormones. Once you have a score, you can do your own math to figure out if the risks and benefits of hormone drugs are worth it to you.

The second Web site, www.yourdisease risk.com, won't give you a score. But it will show you a useful bar graph and where you fall on the risk spectrum, from low to high. You can look at your risk before beginning hormone therapy, then go back and add menopause hormones into your risk profile to see how it changes before and after hormone use.

Regardless of whether a woman uses menopause hormones, she should be getting regular mammograms usually starting at about age 40. Because hormones can change the way a breast appears on a mammogram, a woman who takes estrogen or a combination of estrogen and progestin should talk to her doctor about getting regular breast sonograms as an added precaution.

Osteoporosis

Most medical groups agree that osteoporosis prevention is not a good reason for most women to take menopause hormones. Bone health is one issue that you should consider as you debate the risks and benefits of hormone therapy.

If you suffer from moderate to severe menopausal symptoms and you also are at high risk for bone problems, the benefits of menopause hormones likely outweigh the risks. One analysis of the WHI data showed that among women at high risk for bone problems, using hormones so dramatically lowered their risk of serious fractures that it virtually negated any risks associated with hormone therapy in older women.

The NAMS panel concluded that it's inappropriate to recommend hormone therapy solely for bone preservation, although the panel agreed that low-dose patch treatments are appropriate to help preserve bone health. The ACOG panel says it's appropriate to prescribe menopause hormones to women with osteopenia or osteoporosis.

For women seeking relief from menopause symptoms, it's reasonable to consider the fact that hormone therapy offers bone protection. This and other benefits should be weighed against the risks when making your personal hormone decision.

Mental Health

A woman who takes menopause hormones to relieve menopausal symptoms may notice improvement in her mood as well. Menopause hormones are effective in improving mood and reducing depression. In a large analysis of 38 studies on hormone therapy and mood, reviewers concluded that hormone use produced a 32 percent improvement in mood compared with non-hormone use. Put another way, the women who took hormones were less likely to be depressed than three-quarters of the women who didn't take hormones.[2]

While these data make a strong case for using hormones to improve mood and lower depression during menopause, they also show that some women do just fine without hormone therapy. After all, one in four women who didn't take hormones felt just as well as the women who did take hormones. But clearly, for women with severe mood changes during menopause, hormones are one option for evening out mood swings and avoiding depression.

A review of the medical literature showed that hormone drugs also appear to improve sleep quality in menopausal women.[3] Other studies suggest that menopause hormones may help improve fuzzy thinking, cognitive problems, and executive function in some menopausal women.

Most medical experts don't recommend hormone therapy solely to relieve depressive symptoms or mood issues. Although some studies have found estrogen to have antidepressive effects in perimenopausal women, the ACOG task force recommends trying antidepressant medications first. The task force notes that if you don't want to take antidepressants, or you can't, you might talk with your doctor about estrogen for mild to moderate depression, particularly if you also suffer from hot flashes or other menopause symptoms. Short-term hormone use may help make antidepressants more effective in some women.

Vaginal Dryness/Pain/Sexual Function
Vaginal problems will affect virtually every woman at some point after menopause. If this is the only problem you face, vaginal

estrogen treatments may be enough to ease your symptoms. Women who take menopause hormones to relieve hot flashes and other symptoms will likely experience improvements in vaginal health, a benefit that should be considered along with the other risks and benefits of hormone therapy.

The ACOG task force concluded that there isn't enough evidence for or against the use of estrogen or androgen to improve sex drive in postmenopausal women. However, better vaginal health surely can enhance a woman's sex life after menopause. Some women report an improvement in libido with hormone therapy.

Colon Cancer

Most medical groups don't believe that the protective effect of hormone therapy against colon cancer is great enough to be an important factor in the hormone decision. However, if you have a family history of colon cancer, it may be worthwhile to discuss this issue with your doctor. The ACOG task force notes that, by itself, colon cancer prevention isn't a good reason to start taking menopause hormones. But for a woman with severe menopause symptoms and a family history of colon cancer, hormone therapy might provide some extra protection.

Whatever you decide about menopause hormones, it's important to get a screening colonoscopy at age 50, when colon cancer risk starts to rise.

Special Circumstances

Most of the advice from medical groups about menopause hormones targets women approaching natural menopause who face average health risks. There are some unique situations that deserve attention.

If you're at high risk for breast cancer: Generally, women who have a strong family history of breast cancer or who are breast cancer survivors are advised not to use menopause hormones. For many of these women, alternative treatments such as anti-depressants for hot flashes may provide needed relief. In cases of severe menopause symptoms, some women may opt for low doses of hormones after talking with their doctors about the quality-of-life benefits versus breast cancer risk. Increasingly, doctors are prescribing vaginal estrogen to these women to help with vaginal atrophy. Although the data aren't entirely clear, most doctors believe that vaginal estrogen treatments stay fairly contained in the vagina and that little estrogen ends up circulating in the blood. So these treatments appear to be safe for women with a history of breast cancer or at high risk for the disease.

One important observational study of breast cancer patients, most of whom were taking estrogen alone, reported no increase in recurrence or mortality among women who continued hormone therapy after their diagnosis.[4] Another study of breast cancer patients showed that estrogen users had lower mortality rates from breast cancer than non-estrogen users.[5] So there is still much to be learned about the impact of menopause hormones on women at high risk for breast cancer.

If you're a young woman who has undergone surgical or medical menopause: One of the most frustrating reactions to the WHI is that many young women who undergo surgical removal of their ovaries (surgical menopause) or who lose ovarian function due to medical treatment (medical menopause) are afraid to take menopause hormones. Surgical or medical menopause typically induces far more severe symptoms than natural menopause, but the WHI clearly wasn't designed to answer the types of questions facing these women.

Women who undergo natural menopause are exposed to their own natural estrogen for decades before menopause. However, a woman in her thirties who undergoes surgical menopause is losing out on another 20 years of natural estrogen exposure. For these women, the risk-benefit equation is entirely different. Early research has shown that women who lose ovarian function at a young age appear to be at higher risk for heart problems and osteoporosis if they don't take menopause hormones.

It's important for these women to consider the fact that due to their young age, they are at low risk for the types of health problems (heart attack, stroke, breast cancer) identified in the WHI. So even if they assume the degree of risk found among older women in the WHI, their individual overall risk is so low that hormone use shouldn't have a dramatic impact on their absolute risk.

If you've quit hormones and want to go back on: After the announcement of the WHI results in 2002, scores of women stopped taking menopause hormones overnight. This was definitely an overreaction, and it's a shame that so many women unnecessarily suffered through the effects of quick hormone withdrawal and the return of menopause symptoms. Many of these women weathered the storm and today feel just fine.

But for some women, their menopause symptoms are so potent and persistent that they've not been able to get adequate relief. Now they are wondering if it's too late to resume hormone therapy.

Unfortunately, we don't have an answer to this question. If there is one thing that we learned from the WHI, it's that starting hormone therapy long after menopause — long after the decline of a woman's natural estrogen — is not a good idea. Most of the women in the WHI started taking hormones 10 or more years after menopause. Those who took hormones within 10 years of menopause typically fared better and had fewer serious health problems. For this reason, some doctors now say that a woman who really wants to resume hormone use likely can do so within about 5 years of stopping treatment.

A FINAL WORD ABOUT
YOUR HORMONE DECISION

Now that you know all the facts behind the recent hormone headlines and studies, you should feel well qualified to make your own personal hormone decision. There's a lot to digest and think about, but hopefully, you have come away from this book with a better understanding of the real risks and benefits related to hormone use.

Now that you've done your homework, you should know that there is one important way to eliminate the worry of hormone use. It's exercise.

One of the most compelling scientific findings to come out of the recent hormone debate stems from an analysis of data from both the WHI and the Nurses' Health Study. The aim of this analysis was to compare the younger menopausal women in both studies to see if the data showed similar trends. As you read earlier in this book, researchers found that in both studies, younger women close to menopause appeared to have little increase in risk and likely experienced some protection from hormone use. Women in both studies who began hormone therapy at an older age, long past menopause, appeared to take on far greater risk while gaining fewer benefits.

But in the midst of this analysis, another important finding began to emerge as the researchers turned their attention to the women in both studies who were active and healthy. Among those women, the benefits of a healthy lifestyle were so powerful that they literally erased any impact of menopause hormones. This means that the health gains of exercise and healthful eating far exceed any potential benefit or any potential risk of hormone use. Women in these studies who took hormones and were physically active had the same low risk of health problems as similarly healthy women who opted not to take hormones. It simply didn't matter whether or not these women used hormones. Exercise was more important.

So the most important lesson from years of hormone research may be that regardless of a woman's hormone decision, a healthy lifestyle may be her most important decision of all.

ENDNOTES

Chapter 1

1. Writing Group for the Women's Health Initiative Investigators, "Risks and benefits of estrogen and progestin in healthy post-menopausal women: Principal results form the Women's Health Initiative randomized controlled trial." *JAMA* 288 (2002): 321–333.
2. Seaman, Barbara, *The Greatest Experiment Ever Performed on Women.* (New York: Hyperion, 2003).
3. Rossouw, Jacques, Transcript. Press conference remarks. "Release of the results of the estrogen plus progestin trial of the Women's Health Initiative: Findings and implications." July 9, 2002.
4. Manson, J. E., J. Hsia,, K. C. Johnson, J. E. Rossouw, et al. "Estrogen plus progestin and the risk of coronary heart disease," *New England Journal of Medicine* 349 (2003): 523–534.

5. Hsia, J., R. D. Langer, J. E. Manson, L. Kuller, et al. "Conjugated equine estrogens and coronary heart disease: The Women's Health Initiative." *Archives of Internal Medicine* 166 (2006): 356–365.

6. Stampfer, M. J., W. C. Willett, G. A. Colditz, B. Rosner, F. E. Speizer, and C. H. Hennekens. "A prospective study of postmenopausal estrogen therapy and coronary heart disease in U.S. women." *New England Journal of Medicine* 313 (1985): 1044–1049.

7. Stampfer, M. J., G. A. Colditz, W. C. Willett, J. E. Manson, B. Rosner, F. E. Speizer, and C. H. Hennekens. "Postmenopausal estrogen therapy and cardiovascular disease. Ten-year follow-up from the nurses' health study." *New England Journal of Medicine* 325 (1991): 756–762.

8. Writing Group for the Women's Health Initiative Investigators.

9. The Women's Health Initiative Steering Committee. "Effects of conjugated equine estrogen in postmenopausal women with hysterectomy: The Women's Health Initiative randomized controlled trial." *JAMA* 291 (2004): 1701–1712.

10. Jacques Rossouw. Interview, April 2005.

11. Press release. "NHLBI stops trial of estrogen plus progestin due to increased

breast cancer risk, lack of overall benefit."
National Institutes of Health. July 9, 2002.

12. Hulley, S., D. Grady, T. Bush, C. Furberg, et al. "Randomized trial of estrogen plus progestin for secondary prevention of coronary heart disease in postmenopausal women." *JAMA* 280 (1998): 605–613.

13. Market research data from Wyeth.

14. Haas, J. S., B. Geller, D. L. Miglioretti, D. S. Buist, D. E. Nelson, et al. "Changes in newspaper coverage about hormone therapy with the release of new medical evidence." *Journal of General Internal Medicine* 21(4) (April 2006): 304–309.

15. Press release. "WHI updated analysis: No increased risk of breast cancer with estrogen-alone." National Institutes of Health. April 11, 2006.

Chapter 2

1. Longcope, C. "Endocrine function of the postmenopausal ovary." *Journal of the Society for Gynecologic Investigations* 8(1 Suppl Proceedings) (Jan.–Feb. 2001): S67–68.

2. Ushiroyama, T., O. Sugimoto. "Endocrine function of the peri- and postmenopausal ovary." *Hormone Research* 44(2) (1995): 64–68.

3. Houck, J. A. "How to treat a menopausal

woman: A history, 1900 to 2000." *Current Women's Health Reports* 2 (2002): 349–355.

4. Ibid.

5. Seaman, B. "The history of hormone replacement therapy: A timeline." Kleinman, D. L., A. J. Kinchy, and J. Handelson, eds. *Controversies in Science and Technology: From Maize to Menopause (Science and Technology in Society).* (Madison, WI: University of Wisconsin Press, 2005): 219–235.

6. Houck, J. A. "The medicalization of menopause in America, 1897–2000: Mapping the terrain." Kleinman, D. L., A. J. Kinchy, and J. Handelson, eds. *Controversies in Science and Technology: From Maize to Menopause (Science and Technology in Society).* (Madison, WI: University of Wisconsin Press, 2005): 199–200.

7. Hormone Foundation. The Evolution of Estrogen: A Timeline. www.hormone.org/public/menopause/estrogen_timeline/.

8. Interview with Mike Dey, president of women's health care at Wyeth Pharmaceuticals. Feb 2006.

9. Seaman.

10. Hormone Foundation.

11. Houck (2005)

12. McCrea, F. B. "The politics of meno-

pause: The 'discovery' of a deficiency disease." *Social Problems,* Vol. 31, No. 1 (Oct. 1983): 111–123.

13. Houck, J. A. *Hot and Bothered: Women, Medicine and Menopause in Modern America.* (Cambridge, MA, and London: Harvard University Press, 2006): 152–154.

14. Wilson, M. D., and A. Robert. *Feminine Forever.* (New York: M. Evans and Co., 1996): 15–16.

15. Wilson. p 40.

16. Wilson. p. 67.

17. Wilson. p 206.

18. Houck, J. A. "What do these women want? Feminist responses to *Feminine Forever,* 1963–1980." *Bulletin of the History of Medicine* 77 (2003): 103–132.

19. Cooper, Wendy. *Don't Change: A Biological Revolution for Women.* (New York: Stein and Day, 1975).

20. Houck (2003)

21. Seaman, Barbara. *The Greatest Experiment Ever Performed on Women.* (New York: Hyperion, 2003): 4–6.

22. Seaman.

23. Weiss, N. S., C. L. Ure, J. H. Ballard, A. R. Williams, and J. R. Daling. "Decreased risk of fractures of the hip and

lower forearm with postmenopausal use of estrogen." *N Engl J Med.* 303(21) (Nov. 20, 1980): 1195–1198.

24. Seaman.

25. Stefanick, M. L. "Estrogens and progestins: Background and history, trends in use, and guidelines and regimens approved by the US Food and Drug Administration." *American Journal of Medicine* 188 (2005): 64S–73S.

Chapter 3

1. Avis, N. E., S. L. Crawford, and S. M. McKinlay. "Psychosocial, behavioral, and health factors related to menopause symptomatology." *Women's Health* 3 (1997): 103–120.

2. Freedman, R. R. "Pathophysiology and treatment of menopausal hot flashes." *Seminars in Reproductive Medicine, 23* (2005): 117–125.

3. Freeman, E. W., M. D. Sammel, J. A. Grisso, M. Battistini, et al. "Hot flashes in the late reproductive years: risk factors for African American and Caucasian women." *J Women Health Gend Based Med* 10 (2001): 67–76.

4. Pinkerton, J. V., and A. S. Zion. "Vasomotor symptoms in menopause: Where we've been and where we're going." *Jour-*

nal of Women's Health 15 (2006): 135–145.

5. Freeman.

6. Gold, E. B., B. Sternfeld, J. L. Kelsey, et al. "Relation of demographic and lifestyle factors to symptoms in a multiracial/ethnic population of women 40–55 years of age." Am J Epidemiol 152 (2000): 463–473.

7. Ibid.

8. North American Menopause Society Position Statement. "Treatment of menopause-associated vasomotor symptoms: position statement of the North American Menopause Society." Menopause 11 (2004): 11–33.

9. Ness, J., W. S. Aronow, and G. Beck. "Menopausal symptoms after cessation of hormone replacement therapy." Maturitas (2006): 356–361.

10. Ockene J. K., D. H. Barad, B. B. Cochraine, J. C. Larson, et al. "Symptom experience after discontinuing use of estrogen plus progestin." JAMA 294 (2005): 183–193.

Chapter 4

1. Parker-Pope, T. "Risk of heart attack is greater for women than they realize." Wall Street Journal (June 1, 2001): B1.

2. Grady, D., S. M. Rubin, D. B. Petitti, et al. "Hormone therapy to prevent disease and prolong life in postmenopausal women." *Annals of Internal Medicine* 117 (1992): 1016–1037.

3. Oliver, M., and G. Boyd. "Effect of bilateral ovariectomy on coronary artery disease and serum-lipid levels." *Lancet* 31 (1959): 690–694.

4. Stefanick, M. L. "Estrogens and progestins: Background and history, trends in use, and guidelines and regimens approved by the US Food and Drug Administration." *American Journal of Medicine* Vol. 118(128) (2005): 64S–73S.

5. Bush, T. L., E. Barrett-Connor, L. D. Cowan, et al. "Cardiovascular mortality and noncontraceptive use of estrogen in women: Results from the Lipid Research Clinics program followup study." *Circulation* 75 (1987): 1102–1109.

6. Wilson, P. W., R. J. Garrison, and W. P. Castelli. "Postmenopausal estrogen use, cigarette smoking, and cardiovascular morbidity in women over 50." The Framingham Study.

7. Stampfer, M. J., W. C. Willett, G. A. Colditz, B. Rosner, F. E. Speizer, and C. H. Hennekens. "A prospective study of post-menopausal estrogen therapy and coro-

nary heart disease." (1985).

8. Bush.

9. Petitti, D. B., J. A. Perlman, and S. Sidney. "Noncontraceptive estrogens and mortality: long-term follow-up of women in the Walnut Creek Study." *Obstet Gynecol.* 70(3 Pt 1) (Sept. 1987): 289–293.

10. Stampfer, M. J., G. A. Colditz, W. C. Willett, J. E. Manson, et al. "Postmenopausal estrogen therapy and cardiovascular disease. Ten-year follow-up from the nurses' health study." *N Engl J Med.* 325(11) (Sept. 12, 1991): 756–762.

11. Grady, D., S. M. Rubin, D. B. Petitti, et al. "Hormone therapy to prevent disease and prolong life in postmenopausal women." *Annals of Internal Medicine* 117 (1992): 1016–1037.

12. Barrett-Connor, E., and D. Grady. "Hormone replacement therapy, heart disease, and other considerations." *Annual Review of Public Health* 19 (1998): 55–72.

13. Barrett-Connor, E., and T. L. Bush. "Estrogen and coronary heart disease in women." *JAMA* 265 (1991): 1861–1867.

14. The Writing Group for the PEPI Trial. "Effects of estrogen or estrogen/progestin regimens on heart disease risk factors in postmenopausal women: The Postmenopausal Estrogen/Progestin Interventions

(PEPI) trial." *JAMA* 273 (1995): 199–208.

15. Hulley, S., D. Grady, T. Bush, et al. "Randomized trial of estrogen plus progestin for secondary prevention of coronary heart disease in postmenopausal women." Heart and Estrogen/Progestin Replacement Study (HERS) Research Group. *JAMA* 280(7) (1998): 605–613.

16. Writing group for the Women's Health Initiative. "Risks and benefits of estrogen plus progestin in healthy postmenopausal women: Principal results from the Women's Health Initiative randomized controlled trial." *JAMA* 288 (2002): 321–333.

17. Manson, J. E., J. Hsia, K. C. Johnson, J. E. Rossouw, et al. "Estrogen plus progestin and the risk of coronary heart disease." *NEJM* 349(6) (2003): 523–534.

18. Manson.

19. Hsia, J., R. D. Langer, J. E. Manson, L. Kuller. "Conjugated equine estrogens and coronary heart disease." *Arch Intern Med* 166 (2006): 357–365.

20. Grodstein, F., J. E. Manson, and M. J. Stampfer. "Hormone therapy and coronary heart disease: the role of time since menopause and age at hormone initiation." *J Women's Health* 15(1) (Jan.–Feb. 2006): 35–44.

21. Manson.

22. Hsia.

23. Petersen, A. "Man Who Cloned Cats Has New Cause: Menopausal Women. Mr. Sperling Spends Millions Challenging NIH Study on Hormone Replacement." *Wall Street Journal* (March 22, 2004): page A1.

Chapter 5

1. Feinleib, M. "Breast cancer and artificial menopause: A cohort study." *Journal of the National Cancer Institute* 41 (1968): 315–329.

2. Huang, Z., W. C. Willett, G. A. Colditz, and D. J. Hunter. "Waist circumference, waist:hip ratio, and risk of breast cancer in the Nurses' Health Study." *Am J Epidemiol* 150(12) (1999): 1316–1324.

3. Gammon, M. D., E. M. John, and J. A. Britton. Recreational and occupational physical activities and risk of breast cancer. *J Natl Cancer Inst.* 90(2) (Jan. 21, 1998): 100–117.

4. Seaman, Barbara. *The Greatest Experiment Ever Performed on Women.* (New York: Hyperion, 2003).

5. Rookus, M. A., and F. E. van Leuwen. "Oral contraceptives and risk of breast cancer in women aged 20–54 years." *Lancet* 344 (1994): 844–851.

6. Chlebowski, R. T., S. L. Hendrix, R. D. Langer, M. L. Stefanic. "Influence of estrogen plus progestin on breast cancer and mammography in healthy postmenopausal women: The Women's Health Initiative randomized trial." *JAMA* 289 (2003): 3243–3253.

7. Ibid.

8. Stefanick, M. L., G. L. Anderson, K. L. Margolis, and S. L. Hendrix. "Effects of conjugated equine estrogens on breast cancer and mammography screening in postmenopausal women with hysterectomy." *JAMA* 295 (2006): 1647–1657.

9. Ibid.

10. Kerlikowske, K., D. L. Miglioretti, R. Ballard-Barbash, and D. L. Weaver. "Prognostic characteristics of breast cancer among postmenopausal hormone users in a screened population." *Journal of Clinical Oncology* 21 (2003): 4314–4321.

11. Beral, V., and Million Women Study collaborators. Breast cancer and hormone-replacement therapy in the Million Women Study. *Lancet* 362 (9382) (Aug 9, 2003): 419–427.

12. Feigelson, H. S., E. E. Calle, A. S. Robertson, and P. A. Wingo. "Alcohol consumption increases the risk of fatal breast cancer (United States)." *Cancer Causes*

Control. 12(10) (Dec. 2001): 895–902.

13. Petri, A. L., A. Tjonneland, M. Gamborg, D. Johansen, et al. "Alcohol intake, type of beverage, and risk of breast cancer in pre- and postmenopausal women." *Alcohol Clin Exp Res.* 28(7) (July 2004): 1084–1090.

14. Singletary, K., and S. Gapstur. "Alcohol and breast cancer." *Review of Epidemiologic and Experimental Evidence and Potential Mechanisms. JAMA* 286 (2001): 2143–2151.

15. Mezzetti, M., C. LaVecchia, A. DeCarli, P. Boyle, R. Talamini, and S. Franceschi. "Population attributable risk for breast cancer: diet, nutrition, and physical exercise." *J Natl Cancer Inst.* 90 (1998): 389–394.

16. Chen, W. Y., G. A. Colditz, B. Rosner, S. E. Hankinson, et al. "Use of postmenopausal hormones, alcohol and risk for invasive breast cancer." *Ann Intern Med.* 137(10) (2002): 143.

17. Chen, W. Y., J. E. Manson, S. E. Hankinson, B. Rosner, M. D. Holmes, W. C. Willett, and G. A. Colditz. "Unopposed estrogen therapy and the risk of invasive breast cancer." *Arch Intern Med.* 166(9) (May 8, 2006): 1027–1032.

Chapter 6

1. Kanis, J. A., O. Johnell, C. De Laet, B. Jonsson, et al. "International variations in hip fracture probabilities: implications for risk assessment." *Bone Miner Res.* 17(7) (July 2002): 1237–1244.
2. Cummings, S. R., M. C. Nevitt, W. S. Browner, and K. Stone. "Risk factors for hip fracture in white women." *NEJM* 332 (1995): 767–774.
3. Ibid.
4. Seaman, Barbara. *The Greatest Experiment Ever Performed on Women.* (New York: Hyperion, 2003): 74–75.
5. Seaman, B. "The history of hormone replacement therapy: a timeline." In D. L. Kleinman, A. J. Kinchy, and J. Handelson, eds. *Controversies in Science and Technology: From Maize to Menopause (Science and Technology in Society).* (Madison, WI: University of Wisconsin Press, 2005): 226–227.
6. Cauley, J. A., J. Robbins, Z. Chen, S. R. Cummings, et al. "Effects of estrogen plus progestin on risk of fracture and bone mineral density: the Women's Health Initiative Randomized Trial." *JAMA* 290 (2003): 1729–1738.
7. Jackson, R. D., J. Wactawski-Wende, A. Z. LaCroix, and M. Pettinger. "Effects of

conjugated equine estrogen on risk of fractures and BMD in postmenopausal women with hysterectomy: results from the women's health initiative randomized trial." *J Bone Miner Res.* 21(6) (June 2006): 817–828.

8. Cauley, J. A., J. Robbins, Z. Chen, S. R. Cummings, R. D. Jackson, et al. "Effects of estrogen plus progestin on risk of fracture and bone mineral density: the Women's Health Initiative randomized trial." *JAMA* 290 (2003): 1729–1738.

9. Kuller, L. H., K. A. Matthews, and E. N. Meilahn. "Recency and duration of postmenopausal hormone therapy: effects on bone mineral density and fracture risk in the National Osteoporosis Risk Assessment (NORA) study." *Menopause.* 10(5) (Sept.–Oct. 2003):412–419.

10. Ettinger, B., K. E. Ensrud, R. Wallace, K. C. Johnson, et al. "Effects of ultralow-dose transdermal estradiol on bone mineral density: a randomized clinical trial." *Obstet Gynecol.* 104(3) (Sept. 2004): 443–451.

Chapter 7

1. Woods, N. F., and E. S. Mitchell. "Symptoms during the perimenopause: Prevalence, severity, trajectory, and significance

405

in women's lives." *American Journal of Medicine* 118(12) (2005): 145–245.

2. Bachmann, G. A. "The changes before the 'change': Strategies for the transition to the menopause." *Journal of Postgraduate Medicine* 95 (1994): 113–124.

3. Bachmann, G. A., and S. R. Leiblum. "The impact of hormones on menopausal sexuality: A literature review." *Menopause* 11(1) (2004): 120–130.

4. Graziottin, A., and S. R. Leiblum. "Biological and psychosocial pathophysiology of female sexual dysfunction during the menopausal transition." *Journal of Sexual Medicine* 2 (suppl 3) (2005): 133–143.

5. Goldstein, I., and J. L. Alexander. "Practical aspects in the management of vaginal atrophy and sexual dysfunction in perimenopausal and postmenopausal women." *Journal of Sexual Medicine* 2(suppl 3) (2005): 154–165.

6. Alexander, J. L., K. Kotz, L. Dennerstein, S. J. Kutner, et al. The effects of postmenopausal hormone therapies on female sexual functioning: A review of double-blind, randomized controlled trials." *Menopause* 11(6) (2004): 749–765.

7. Gorodeski, G. I. "Effects of estrogen on proton secretion via the apical membrane

in vaginal-ectocervical epithelial cells of postmenopausal women." *Menopause* 12 (2005): 679–684.

8. Bachmann, G. "Quantifying estrogen treatment effect on vagina tissue: Cellular age matters." *Menopause* 12(6) (2005): 656–657.

9. Bachmann, G. A., and S. R. Leiblum. "The impact of hormones on menopausal sexuality: A literature review." *Menopause* 11(1) (2004): 120–130.

10. Leiblum, S., G. Bachmann, E. Kemmann, D. Colburn, and L. Swartzman. "Vaginal atrophy in the postmenopausal woman: The importance of sexual activity and hormones." *JAMA* 249(16) (1983): 2195–2198.

11. Dennerstein, L., P. Lehert, and H. Burger. "The relative effects of hormones and relationship factors on sexual function of women through the natural menopausal transition." *Fertility and Sterility* 84 (2005): 174–180.

12. Addis, I. B., S. K. Van Den Eeden, C. L. Wassel-Fyr, et al. "Sexual activity and function in middle-aged and older women." *Obstetrics & Gynecology* 107 (2006): 755–764.

13. Dennerstein, L., and P. Lehert. "Modeling mid-aged women's sexual functioning:

A prospective population-based study." *Journal of Sex & Marital Therapy* 30 (2004): 173–183.

14. Ibid.

15. "Menopause — Myths and Medicine." Quantum. Australian Broadcasting Corp. Original broadcast June 22, 2000. (Transcript at www.abc.net.au/quantum/stories/s140519.htm).

16. Dennerstein, L., J. Randolph, J. Taffe, E. Dudley, and H. Burger. "Hormones, mood, sexuality and the menopausal transition." *Fertility and Sterility* 77(4) (2002): S42–S48.

17. Dennerstein, L., E. Dudley, and H. Burger. "Are changes in sexual functioning during midlife due to aging or menopause?" *Fertility and Sterility* 76 (2001): 456–460.

18. Ibid.

19. Dennerstein, L. "Depressed libido in the postmenopausal woman." Medscape Ask the Experts (online). Cited February 12, 2003. (www.medscape.com/viewarticle/448554_print).

20. Alexander, et al.

21. Ibid.

22. North American Menopause Society. "The role of testosterone therapy in postmenopausal women: Position statement of

the North American Menopause Society." *Menopause* 12 (2005): 497–511.

23. Dennerstein, L., J. Randolph, J. Taffe, E. Dudley, and H. Burger. "Hormones, mood, sexuality and the menopausal transition." *Fertility and Sterility* 77(4) (2002): S42–S48.

24. Ibid.

25. Ibid.

26. Davis, S. R., S. L. Davison, S. Donath, and R. Bell. "Relationships between circulating androgen levels and self-reported sexual function in women." *JAMA* 294 (2005): 91–96.

27. *Wall Street Journal* citation.

28. NAMS position statement.

Chapter 8

1. Yaffe, K., G. Sawaya, I. Lieberburg, and D. Grady. "Estrogen therapy in postmenopausal women: Effects on cognitive function and dementia." *JAMA* 279 (1998): 699–695.

2. Benes, F. M., M. Turtle, Y. Khan, and P. Farol. "Myelination of a key relay zone in the hippocampal formation occurs in the human brain during childhood, adolescence, and adulthood." Arch Gen Psychiatry 51(6) (June 1994): 477–484.

3. Meyer, P. M., L. H. Powell, R. S. Wilson,

et al. "A population-based longitudinal study of cognitive functioning in the menopausal transition." *Neurology* 61 (2003): 801–806.

4. Ibid.

5. Henderson, V. W., J. R. Guthrie, E. C. Dudley, H. G. Burger, et al. "Estrogen exposures and memory at midlife: A population-based study of women." *Neurology* 60 (2003): 1369–1371.

6. Mitchell, E. S. and N. F. Woods. "Midlife women's attributions about perceived memory changes: Observations from the Seattle Midlife Women's Health Study." *Journal of Women's Health and Gender-Based Medicine* 10 (2001): 351–362.

7. Gold, E. B., B. Sternfeld, J. L. Kelsey, et al. "Relation of demographic and lifestyle factors to symptoms in a multi-racial/ethnic population of women 40–55 years of age." *American Journal of Epidemiology* 152 (2000): 463–473.

8. LeBlanc, E. S., J. Janowsky, B. Chan, H. D. Nelson. "Hormone replacement therapy and cognition: Systematic review and meta-analysis." *JAMA* 285 (2001): 1489–1499.

9. Shaywitz, S. E., F. Naftolin, D. Phil, D. Zelterman, et al. "Better oral reading and short-term memory in midlife, post-

menopausal women taking estrogen." *Menopause* 10(5) (2003): 420–426.

10. Joffe, H., J. E. Hall, S. Gruber, I. A. Sarmiento, et al. "Estrogen therapy selectively enhances prefrontal cognitive processes: a randomized, double-blind, placebo-controlled study with functional magnetic resonance imaging in perimenopausal and recently postmenopausal women." *Menopause* 13(3) (May–June 2006): 411–422.

11. Zandi, P. P., et al. "Hormone replacement therapy and incidence of Alzheimer's disease in older women: The Cache County Study." *JAMA* 288 (2002): 2123–2129.

12. Yaffe, K., G. Sawaya, I. Lieberburg, and D. Grady. "Estrogen therapy in postmenopausal women: Effects on cognitive function and dementia." *JAMA* 279(9) (1998): 688–695.

13. LeBlanc, E. S., J. Janowsky, B. K. Chan, and H. D. Nelson. "Hormone replacement therapy and cognition: Systemic review and meta-analysis." *JAMA* 285(11) (2001): 1489–1499.

14. Shumaker, S. A., C. Legault, L. Kuller, et al. "Conjugated equine estrogens and incidence of probable dementia and mild cognitive impairment in postmenopausal

women: Women's Health Initiative Memory Study." *JAMA* 291 (2004): 2947–2958.

15. Ibid.

16. Breitner, J., and P. P. Zandi. "Effects of estrogen plus progestin on risk of dementia." *JAMA* 290 (2003): 1706.

17. Bagger, Y. Z., L. B. Tanko, P. Alexandersen, et al. "Early postmenopausal hormone therapy may prevent cognitive impairment later in life." *Menopause* 12(1) (2005): 12–17.

18. MacLennan, A. H., V. W. Henderson, B. J. Paine, et al. "Hormone therapy, timing of initiation, and cognition in women aged older than 60 years: The REMEMBER pilot study." *Menopause* 13(1) (2006): 28–36.

19. Dell, D. L., and D. E. Stewart. "Menopause and mood: Is depression linked with hormone changes?" *Postgraduate Medicine* 180(3) (2000).

20. Avis, N. E., D. Brambilla, S. M. McKinlay, et al. "A longitudinal analysis of the association between menopause and depression: Results from the Massachusetts Women's Health Study." *Annals of Epidemiology* 4(3) (1994): 214–220.

21. Bromberger, J. T., S. F. Assmann, N. E. Avis, et al. "Persistent mood symptoms in

412

a multiethnic community cohort of pre- and peri-menopausal women." *American Journal of Epidemiology* 158 (2003): 347–356.

22. Cohen, L. S., C. N. Soares, A. F. Vitonis, et al. "Risk for new onset of depression during the menopausal transition." *Archives of General Psychiatry* 63 (2006): 385–390.

23. Freeman, E. W., M. D. Sammel, H. Lin, and D. B. Nelson. "Associations of hormones and menopausal status with depressed mood in women with no history of depression." *Archives of General Psychiatry* 63(4) (Apr 2006): 375–382.

24. Zweifel, J. E., and W. H. O'Brien. "A meta-analysis of the effect of hormone replacement therapy upon depressed mood." *Psychoneuroendocrinology* 22(3) (1997): 189–212.

25. Woods, N. F., and Mitchell E. Sullivan. "Symptoms during the perimenopause: Prevalence, severity, trajectory and significance in women's lives." *American Journal of Medicine* 118(128) (2005): 145–245.

26. Shaver, J., and S. N. Zenk. "Sleep disturbance in menopause." *Journal of Women's Health & Gender-Based Medicine* 9(2) (2000): 109–118.

27. Antonijevic, I. A., G. K. Stalla, A. Steiger. "Modulation of the sleep electroencephalogram by estrogen replacement in postmenopausal women." *American Journal of Obstetrics and Gynecology* 182 (2000):277–282.

28. Brunner, R. L., M. Gass, A. Aragaki, J. Hays, et al. "Effects of conjugated equine estrogen on health-related quality of life in postmenopausal women with hysterectomy: Results from the Women's Health Initiative randomized clinical trial." *Archives of Internal Medicine* 165 (2005): 1976–1986.

29. Bushnell, C. D. "Hormone replacement therapy and stroke: The current state of knowledge and directions for future research." *Seminars in Neurology* 26(1) (2006): 123–130.

30. Wassertheil-Smoller, S., S. L. Hendrix, M. Limacher, G. Heiss, et al. "Effect of estrogen plus progestin on stroke in postmenopausal women: The Women's Health Initiative: A randomized trial." *JAMA* 289 (2003): 2673–2684.

31. Hendrix, S. L., S. Wassertheil-Smoller, K. C. Johnson, and B. V. Howard. "Effects of conjugated equine estrogen on stroke in the Women's Health Initiative." *Circulation* 113 (2006): 2425–2434.

32. Thomas, T., N. Haase, W. Rosamond, et al. "Heart disease and stroke statistics — 2006 update: A report from the American Heart Association statistics committee and stroke statistics subcommittee." *Circulation* (Feb. 2006).

Chapter 9

1. Brincat, M., S. Kabalan, J. W. Studd, et al. "A study of the decrease of skin collagen content, skin thickness, and the bone mass in the postmenopausal woman." *Obstetrics and Gynecology* 70 (1987): 840–845.
2. Brincat, M. P., Baron Y. Muscat, and R. Galea. "Estrogens and the skin." *Climacteric* 8 (2005): 110–123.
3. Verdier-Sevrain, S., F. Bonte, and B. Gilchrest. "Biology of estrogens in skin: Implications for skin aging." *Experimental Dermatology* 15 (2006): 83–94.
4. Draelos, Z. D. "Topical and oral estrogens revisited for antiaging purposes." *Fertility and Sterility* 84 (2005): 291–292.
5. Brincat, M., S. Kabalan, J. W. Studd, et al. "A study of the decrease of skin collagen content, skin thickness, and the bone mass in the postmenopausal woman." *Obstetrics and Gynecology* 70 (1987): 840–845.

6. Maheux, R., et al. "A randomized, double-blind, placebo-controlled study on the effect of conjugated estrogens on skin thickness." *American Journal of Obstetrics and Gynecology* 170(2) 91994): 642–649.

7. Chen, L., M. Dyson, J. Rymer, et al. "The use of high-frequency diagnostic ultrasound to investigate the effect of hormone replacement therapy on skin thickness." *Skin Research and Technology* 7 (2001): 95–97.

8. Fuchs, K. O., O. Solis, R. Tapawan, and J. Paranjpe. "The effects of an estrogen and glycolic acid cream on the facial skin of postmenopausal women: a randomized histologic study." *Cutis* 71(6) (2003): 481–488.

9. Dunn, L. B., M. Damesyn, A. A. Moore, et al. "Does estrogen prevent skin aging? Results from the First National Health and Nutrition Examination Survey (NHANES I)." *Archives of Dermatology* 133(11) (1997): 1460–1462.

10. Castelo-Branco, C., F. Figueras, M. J. Martinez de Osaba, and J. A. Vanrell. "Facial wrinkling in postmenopausal women. Effects of smoking status and hormone replacement therapy." *Maturitas* 29(1) (1998): 75–86.

11. Creidi, P., B. Faivre, P. Agache, et al.

"Effect of a conjugated oestrogen (Premarin) cream on aging facial skin. A comparative study with a placebo cream." *Maturitas* 19(3) (1994): 211–223.

12. Schmidt, J. B., M. Binder, G. Demschik, et al. "Treatment of skin aging with topical estrogens." *International Journal of Dermatology* 35(9) (1996): 669–674.

13. Wolff, E. F., D. Narayan, H. S. Taylor. "Long-term effects of hormone therapy on skin rigidity and wrinkles." *Fertility and Sterility* 84 (2005): 285–288.

14. Baumann, L. "A dermatologist's opinion on hormone therapy and skin aging." *Fertility and Sterility* 84 (2005): 289–290.

15. Chen, L. M. Dyson, J. Rymer, et al. "The use of high-frequency diagnostic ultrasound to investigate the effect of hormone replacement therapy on skin thickness." *Skin Research and Technology* 7 (2001): 95–97.

16. Draelos, Z. D. "Topical and oral estrogens revisited for antiaging purposes." *Fertility and Sterility* 84 (2005): 291–292.

17. Brincat, M. P., Baron Y. Muscat, and R. Galea. "Estrogens and the skin." *Climacteric* 8 (2005): 110–123.

Chapter 10

1. American Cancer Society Cancer Statistics 2006. Estimated new cancer cases and deaths by sex, for all sites. US, 2006.

2. Chlebowski, R. T., J. Wactawski-Wende, C. Ritenbaugh, and F. A. Hubbell. "Estrogen plus progestin and colorectal cancer in postmenopausal women." *N Engl J Med.* 350(10) (March 4, 2004): 991–1004.

3. Coughlin, S. S., A. Giustozzi, S. J. Smith, and N. C. Lee. "A meta-analysis of estrogen replacement therapy and risk of epithelial ovarian cancer." *J Clin Epidemiol.* 53 (2000): 367–375.

4. Garg, P. P., K. Kerlikowske, L. Subak, and D. Grady. "Hormone replacement therapy and the risk of epithelial ovarian carcinoma: a meta-analysis." *Obstet Gynecol.* 92 (1998): 472–479.

5. Lacey, J. V., P. J. Mink, J. H. Lubin, M. E. Sherman, et al. "Menopausal hormone replacement therapy and risk of ovarian cancer." *JAMA* 288 (2002): 334–341.

6. Moehrer, B., A. Hextall, and S. Jackson. "Oestrogens for urinary incontinence in women" (abstract). *Cochrane Database Syst Rev.* Available at www.update-software.com/abstracts/ab001405.htm.

7. DuBeau, C. E. "Estrogen treatment for urinary incontinence: Now, never or in

the future?" *JAMA* 293 (2005): 998–1001.

8. Hendrix, S. L., B. B. Cochrane, I. E. Nygaard, V. L. Handa, et al. "Effects of estrogen with and without progestin on urinary incontinence." *JAMA* 293(8) (Feb. 23, 2005): 935–948.

9. DuBeau, C. E. "Estrogen treatment for urinary incontinence: Now, never or in the future?" *JAMA* 293 (2005): 998–1001.

10. Hulley, S., C. Furberg, E. Barrett-Connor, et al. "Noncardiovascular disease outcomes during 6.8 years of hormone therapy." *The Journal of the American Medical Association* 288 (2002): 58–66.

11. Simon, J. A., D. B. Hunninghake, S. K. Agarwal, et al. "Effect of estrogen plus progestin on risk for biliary tract surgery in menopausal women with coronary artery disease." The Heart and Estrogen/ Progestin Replacement Study. *Annals of Internal Medicine* 135 (2001): 493–501.

12. Utian, W. H., M. L. Gass, and J. H. Pickar. "Body mass index does not influence response to treatment, nor does body weight change with lower doses of conjugated estrogens and medroxyprogesterone acetate in early postmenopausal women." *Menopause* 11(3) (May–June 2004): 306–314.

13. Barnabei, V. M., B. B. Cochraine, A. K.

Aragaki, I. Nygaard, et al. "Menopausal symptoms and treatment-related effects of estrogen and progestin in the Women's Health Inititaive." *Obstetrics & Gynecology* 105 (2005): 1063–1073.

14. Hunt, B. E., J. A. Taylor, J. W. Hamner, et al. "Estrogen replacement therapy improves baroreflex regulation of vascular sympathetic outflow in postmenopausal women." *Circulation* 103 (2001): 2909–2914.

15. Wyss, J. M., and S. H. Carlson. "Effects of hormone replacement therapy on the sympathetic nervous system and blood pressure." *Curr Hypertens Rep.* 5(3) (June 2003): 241–246.

16. Thunell, L., E. Stadberg, I. Milsom, and L. A. Mattsson. "A longitudinal population study of climacteric symptoms and their treatment in a random sample of Swedish women." *Climacteric* 7(4) (Dec. 2004): 357–365.

17. Sowers, M. R., D. McConnell, M. Jannausch, et al. "Estradiol and its metabolites and their association with knee osteoarthritis." *Arthritis Rheum.* 54(8) (July 26, 2006): 2481–2487.

18. Barnabei, et al.

19. Bonds, D. E., N. Lasser, L. Qi, R. Brzyski, et al. "The effect of conjugated

equine oestrogen on diabetes incidence: the Women's Health Initiative randomized trial." *Diabetologia.* 49 (2006): 459–468.

Chapter 11

1. Harris, V., A. L. Sandridge, R. J. Black, D. H. Brewster, and A. Gould. "Cancer registration statistics Scotland 1986–1995." (Edinburgh: ISD Scotland Publications, 1998.) [cited 14 May 2002].
2. Ries, L. A. G., D. Harkins, M. Krapcho, A. Mariotto, B. A. Miller, E. J. Feuer, L. Clegg, M. P. Eisner, M. J. Horner, N. Howlader, M. Hayat, B. F. Hankey, and B. K. Edwards, eds. *SEER Cancer Statistics Review, 1975–2003,* National Cancer Institute. Bethesda, MD, http:// seer.cancer.gov/csr/1975_2003/, based on November 2005 SEER data submission, posted to the SEER Web site 2006.
3. Murphy, S. J., R. J. Traystman, and P. D. Hurn. "Progesterone exacerbates striatal stroke injury in progesterone-deficient female animals." *Stroke* 31 (2000): 1173.
4. The Writing Group for the PEPI Trial. "Effects of estrogen or estrogen/progestin regimens on heart disease risk factors in postmenopausal women." *JAMA* 273(3) (1995): 199–208.
5. Lakoski, S. G., B. Brosnihan, and D. M.

Herrington. "Hormone therapy, C-reactive protein, and progression of atherosclerosis: data from the Estrogen Replacement on Progression of Coronary Artery Atherosclerosis (ERA) trial." *American Heart Journal* 150(5) (Nov 2005): 907–911.

6. Schairer, C. "Progesterone receptors — animal models and cell signaling in breast cancer: Implications for breast cancer of inclusion of progestins in hormone replacement therapies." *Breast Cancer Research* 4(6) (2002): 244–248.

7. Hofseth, L. J., A. M. Raafat, J. R. Osuch, D. R. Pathak, C. A. Slomski, and S. Z. Haslam. "Hormone replacement therapy with estrogen or estrogen plus medroxyprogesterone acetate is associated with increased epithelial proliferation in the normal postmenopausal breast." *Journal of Clinical Endocrinology & Metabolism* 84 (1999): 4559–4565.

8. Schairer.

9. Writing Group for the PEPI Trial.

10. Persson, I., E. Thurfjell, and L. Holmberg. "Effect of estrogen and estrogen-progestin replacement regimens on mammographic breast parenchymal density." *Journal of Clinical Oncology* 15 (1997): 3201–3207.

11. Lundström, E., B. Wilczek, Z. von Palffy, G. Söderqvist, and B. von Schoultz. "Mammographic breast density during hormone replacement therapy: Differences according to treatment." *American Journal of Obstetrics & Gynecology* 181 (1999): 348–352.

12. Prestwood, K. M., A. M. Kenny, A. Kleppinger, and M. Kulldorff. "Ultralow-dose micronized 17-beta-estradiol and bone density and bone metabolism in older women: a randomized controlled trial." *JAMA* 290(8) (Aug. 27, 2003): 1042–1048

13. Ettinger, B., K. E. Ensrud, R. Wallace, K. C. Johnson, et al. "Effects of ultralow-dose transdermal estradiol on bone mineral density: a randomized clinical trial." *Obstet Gynecol* 104(3) (Sep. 2004): 443–451.

Chapter 12

1. Million Women Study Collaborators. "Breast cancer and hormone replacement therapy in the Million Women Study." *Lancet* 362 (2003): 419–427.

2. Smith, N. L., S. R. Heckbert, R. N. Lemaitre, et al. "Esterified estrogens and conjugated equine estrogens and the risk of venous thrombosis." *JAMA* 292 (2004):

1581–1587.

3. Ibid.

4. Friebely, J. S., J. L. Shifren, I. Schiff, and Q. R. Regestein. "Preliminary observations on differing psychological effects of conjugated and esterified estrogen treatments." *Journal of Women's Health & Gender-Based Medicine* 10 (2001): 181–187.

5. Smith, et al.

6. Tamimi, R. M., S. E. Hankinson, W. Y. Chen, et al. "Combined estrogen and testosterone use and risk of breast cancer in postmenopausal women." *Archives of Internal Medicine* 166 (2006): 1483–1489.

7. Boothby, L. A., P. L. Doering, and S. Kipersztok. "Bioidentical hormone therapy: A review." *Menopause* 11(3) (2004): 356–357.

8. Boothby.

Chapter 13

1. Carroll, D. G. "Nonhormonal therapies for hot flashes in menopause." *American Family Physician* 73 (2006): 457-464, 467.

2. Wutke, W., D. Seidlova-Wutke, and C. Gorkow. "The cimicfuga preparation BNO 1055 vs. conjugated estrogens in a double-blind placebo-controlled study; effects on menopause symptoms and bone

markers." *Maturitas* 44(suppl 1) (2003): 567–577.

3. Scambia, G., D. Mango, P. G. Signorile, et al. "Clinical effects of a standardized soy extract in postmenopausal women: A pilot study." *Menopause* 7 (2000): 105–111.

4. Upmalis, D. H., R. Lobo, L. Bradle, et al. "Vasomotor symptom relief by soy isoflavone extract tablets in postmenopausal women: A multicenter, double-blind randomized placebo-controlled study." *Menopause* 7 (2000): 236–243.

5. Faure, E., P. Chantre, and P. Mares. "Effects of a standardized soy extract on hot flashes, a multicenter, double-blind randomized placebo controlled study." *Menopause* 9 (2002): 329–334.

6. Carroll, D. G. "Nonhormonal therapies for hot flashes in menopause." *American Family Physician* 73 (2006): 457–464, 467.

7. Penotti, M., E. Fabio, A. B. Modena, et al. "Effect of soy-derived isoflavones on hot flushes, endometrial thickness and the pulsatility index of the uterine and cerebral arteries." *Fertility & Sterility* 79 (2003): 1112–1117.

8. Van de Weijer, P. H., and R. Barentsen. "Isoflavones from red clover significantly reduce menopausal hot flush symptoms

compared with placebo." *Maturitas* 42 (2002): 187–193.

9. Carroll.

10. Nelson, H. D., K. K. Vesco, E. Haney, et al. "Nonhormonal therapies for menopausal hot flashes: Systematic review and meta-analysis." *JAMA* 295(17) (2006): 2057–2071.

11. Ibid.

12. Dorsey, C. M., K. A. Lee, and M. B. Scharf. "Effect of zolpidem on sleep in women with perimenopausal and postmenopausal insomnia: A 4-week, randomized, multicenter, double-blind, placebo-controlled study." *Clinical Therapeutics* 10 (2004): 1578–1586.

13. Leiblum, S., G. A. Bachmann, E. Kemmann, D. Colburn, and L. Swartzman. "Vaginal atrophy and the postmenopausal women: The importance of sexual activity and hormones." *JAMA* 249 (1983): 2195–2198.

14. Bygdeman, M., and M. L. Swahn. "Replens versus dienoestrol cream in the symptomatic treatment of vaginal atrophy in postmenopausal women." *Maturitas* 23 (1996): 259–263.

15. Willhite, L. A., and M. O'Connell. "Urogenital atrophy: Prevention and treatment." *Pharmacotherapy* 21(4) (2001):

464–480.

16. North American Menopause Society. "Management of osteoporosis in post-menopausal women: 2006 position statement of the North American Menopause Society." *Menopause* 13 (2006): 340–367.

17. Kanis, J. A., H. Johansson, O. Johnell, et al. "Alcohol intake as a risk factor for fracture." *Osteoporosis International* 16 (2005): 737–742.

18. NAMS position statement.

Chapter 14

1. Minelli, C., K. R. Abrams, A. J. Sutton, and N. J. Cooper. "Benefits and harms associated with hormone replacement therapy: Clinical decision analysis." *BMJ.* 328(7436) (2004): 371.

2. Zweifel, J. E., and W. H. O'Brien. "A meta-analysis of the effect of hormone replacement therapy upon depressed mood." *Psychoneuroendocrinology* 22(3) (1997): 189–212.

3. Shaver, J., and S. N. Zenk. "Sleep disturbance in menopause." *Journal of Women's Health & Gender-Based Medicine* 9(2) (2000): 109–118.

4. O'Meara, E. S., M. A. Rossing, J. R. Daling, et al. "Hormone replacement therapy after a diagnosis of breast cancer in rela-

tion to recurrence and mortality." *Journal of the National Cancer Institute* 93(10) (2001): 754–762.

5. Schairer, C., M. Gail, C. Byrne, et al. "Estrogen replacement therapy and breast cancer survival in a large screening study." *Journal of the National Cancer Institute* 91(3) (1999): 264–270.

ACKNOWLEDGMENTS

Ever since the first results from the Women's Health Initiative (WHI) were announced, I've received endless questions from women who were trying to make sense of this confusing but important study. I am especially grateful to those readers who have openly shared their personal health experiences. Their intelligence and thoughtfulness have inspired me to keep asking better questions and were the impetus for this book.

I am indebted to the many investigators who worked on the Women's Health Initiative — researchers whose contributions have forever changed the course of women's health. Stanford University School of Medicine professor Marcia Stefanick, PhD, who heads the WHI steering committee, deserves special mention for the many hours she has spent discussing the complexities of the WHI. She aptly notes that "science doesn't always work in sound bites," but she has done her best to make the details of this complicated research accessible to the rest of us. I'd also like to thank WHI investigators JoAnn Manson, MD, of Harvard Medical School; Ross Prentice, PhD, and Andrea LaCroix, PhD, both from the University of Washington; and Rowan Chlebowski, MD, from the University of California, Los Angeles — all of whom always managed to make time for my questions. Jacques Rossouw, MD, of the National Institutes of Health suffered a great deal of criticism for his role in the WHI, but I have found him to be a committed, passionate scientist who has been unwavering in his beliefs. I'd also like to thank Wulf Utian, MD, executive director of the North American Menopause Society, who has shared his insights and experiences from both patients and other physicians trying to reconcile long-held beliefs with WHI findings. I've especially enjoyed getting to know Barbara Seaman, who not only has personally chronicled the history of women's health but also, through her writings and activism, has changed the course of it.

My editors and colleagues at the *Wall Street Journal* have given me the space, time, and guidance needed to keep writing about women, menopause, and hormones. I am especially grateful to my good friend Larry Rout, who not only allowed me to write about rethinking the WHI in a special *Wall Street Journal* report in 2003 but also channeled his inner menopausal woman to give me much-needed advice about my manuscript. My agent, Binky Urban, convinced me there was a need for this book, and I appreciate her continued support. Thanks also to Heather Jackson, Susan Berg, and all the people at Rodale who scrambled to make this book happen even as death, divorce, illness, work deadlines, and Delaware River flooding conspired against us.

I am grateful every day for the great women in my life: my sister Liani, who kept me going after the death of my mom; my clever friend Lynn, who came up with the title and who knows far too much about me and remains my friend anyway; my colleague and friend Laura Landro, my own personal guardian angel who has given me needed perspective about life, health, and family relationships; Roxanne, whom I can always count on for anything and everything; Grace, who is just Grace, and that's more than enough; of course, Jane, the unsung hero of my life, whose friendship, advice, and support sustain me; and her special daughters, Arleigh, who can always remember the things I forget, and Ashleigh, who always makes me smile.

And finally, I want to thank my daughter, Laney, who brings me so much joy and makes every moment worthwhile. I am proud of you every day and am so lucky to be your mom.

INDEX

A

Acetylcholine, 209

Aches, body, hormone therapy and, 269–70

Acne, testosterone and, 201

ACOG, 325, 370–84

Activella, 309–10, 314

Actonel, 353

Age. *See also* Older women

  bone loss and, 162–64

  brain function and, 205–15

  breast cancer incidence by, 129, 137

  incontinence and, 262–63

  osteoporosis and, 167–69

  WHI study and, 21–24, 29–34, 111–18

Agrimony, for vaginal dryness, 348

Albright, Fuller, 173, 243–44

Alcohol consumption

  breast cancer risk and, 154–56

  fracture risk and, 349

  hot flashes and, 371

  sleep and, 233, 343

B

Baltimore Longitudinal Study of Aging, 222
Baumann, Leslie, 251
Biest compounded hormones, 321
Bio-identical hormones. *See* Compounded hormones
Birth control pills
  blood pressure and, 329
  breast cancer risk and, 136–37
  colon cancer and, 257
  endometrial cancer and, 330–31
  gallbladder disease and, 266
  heart attacks and, 330
  in history, 69
  ovarian cancer and, 259, 330–31
  progestin as, 279
  smoking and, 329
  strength of hormones in, 329
  stroke and, 235
Bisphosphonates, 180, 353–55
Black cohosh
  bone health and, 352
  hot flashes and, 336
  sleep and, 345
  vaginal dryness and, 348
Bladder control. *See* Incontinence
Blood clots
  ACOG advice, 372–74
  causes of, 372

British Medical Journal study, 362

C

Caffeine
  bone health and, 170
  hot flashes and, 371
  sleep and, 233, 343
Calcimar, 356
Calcitonin, 356
Calcium supplements, 180, 349–51
Cancer. *See specific types*
Cenestin, 308, 316
Chamomile, sleep and, 345
Chaste tree, vaginal dryness and, 348
Cholesterol
  estrogen and, 105, 108–9, 121–23
  gallbladder disease and, 265–66
  hormone use when high, 121–22
  in menopausal women, 104–5
  statins and, 123
  stroke risk and, 376
Chrohn's disease, gallbladder and, 265–66
Climara, 310–11, 312, 314
Clonidine, 342
Coffee. *See* Caffeine
Cognition. *See also* Memory
  aging and, 205–9
  estrogen and, 209–21
  fuzzy thinking, 82, 200, 382
  hormone therapy and, 382

Cycrin, 312–13

D

Decision-making criteria
family health history, 368–69
health assessment, 367–68
side effects, 366–67
symptoms assessment, 363–66
Dehydroepiandrosterone (DHEA), 195,
321
Dementia
age and incidence of, 204
hormone therapy and, 204, 222–23,
226–28, 237
Dennerstein, Lorraine, 185–86, 191–92
Depo Provera, 288
Depression
antidepressants and, 382
hormone therapy and, 205, 230, 237, 382
as menopause symptom, 82, 228
non-hormone therapy for, 238
during perimenopause, 229
DES, 58, 134–35
DHEA, 195, 321
Diabetes
complications from, 271
endometrial cancer risk and, 282–83
as heart disease risk factor, 123
hormone therapy and, 271–72
research findings, 271–72

E

Eating binges, as menopause symptom, 83

Effexor, 340

Emmenin oral estrogen, 57–58

Emotions, antidepressants and, 341

Endometrial cancer. *See* Uterine cancer

Enjuvia, 308

Epilepsy, progestin and, 284

ERA study, 285

Esterified estrogens/testosterone treatment, 308–9, 315–16

Estinyl, 310, 316

Estrace, 309–10, 316, 321

Estraderm patch, 310–11

Estradiol

  in compounded hormones, 320

  decline of

    sexual dysfunction and, 192

    vaginal symptoms and, 185

  effects of progestin on, 281

  forms of

    acetate, 310

    face cream, 247

    generic, 309–10

    micronized, 296

    patches, 310–11

  origins of, 78

Estratab, 308–9

Estratest, 198, 308–9, 315–16

Estring vaginal ring, 316–17

                    448

L

Language skills, estrogen and, 218
LDL cholesterol
  of hormone users, heart risks and,
    122–23
  in menopausal women, 104–5
Levonorgestrel, 289, 314
LH. *See* Luteinizing hormone
Libido, in menopause, 84
Life expectancy, 52
Lifestyle changes
  for bone health, 348–49
  for heart health, 102, 124–25
  for hot flashes, 334–35
  importance of, to overall health, 388–89
  to improve health, 333–34
  for sleep problems, 342–44
  for vaginal dryness, 346–47
Lipid Research Clinics Followup, 105–6
Lobular cancer, 148
Love, Susan, 146
Low-density lipoproteins. *See* LDL
    cholesterol
Lubricants, vaginal, 187, 189, 202, 347–48
Lunesta, 346
Lupron, 210
Luteinizing hormone (LH)
  black cohosh and, 337
  function of, in body, 78–79

454

compared to micronized progesterone, 290

as treatment choice, 312–13

WHI concerns about safety of, 312–13

Myelination, in brain, 206–7

N

NAMS, 52–53, 197, 199–201, 325, 370

National Health and Nutrition Examination Survey (NHANES 1), 248

National Heart, Lung and Blood Institute (NHLBI), 25, 37, 39–40, 149

National Institutes of Health, 28, 46, 49

National Osteoporosis Foundation, 167

National Women's Health Network, 70

Neurontin, 342

NHANES 1 survey, 248

NHLBI, 25, 37, 39–40, 149

Night sweats
  ACOG advice, 371
  hormone therapy for, 371
  lifestyle changes and, 333–34, 371
  as menopause symptom, 81
  sleep and, 231

Norepinephrine
  in brain, estrogen and, 209
  role in hot flashes, 90

Norethindrone acetate, 289, 314

Norgestimate, 289, 314, 329

North American Menopause Society
(NAMS), 52–53, 197, 199–201, 325,
370
Nurses' Health Study
findings of, about
breast cancer risk, 131–32, 138, 155,
160–61, 200, 316, 377
gallbladder disease, 266
heart attacks, 26–28, 105–6
origins of, 70
reservations about, 26–27
testosterone and, 201
WHI study and, 44, 118–21

O

Obesity
bone health and, 170
breast cancer risk and, 132–33, 152
endometrial cancer risk and, 282
gallbladder disease and, 265–66
heart disease risk and, 123–24
Ogen, 310, 316
Older women
bone loss and, 162–81
heart disease as killer of, 99
hormone therapy and
breast cancer risk and, 138–39
cognition and, 204–5
dementia and, 222–23

weight loss and, 91

Testosterone

fatigue and, 84

patch, in development, 197

potential effects of, 199–201

produced by ovaries, 195

sexual health and, 195–98

testing, for women, 198–99

Thermoneutral zone, 90

Thinking, fuzzy

hormone therapy and, 237, 382

as menopause symptom, 82

testosterone and, 200

Timing of hormone use

for cognitive function, 226

for heart health, 111–18, 375

Triest compounded hormones, 321

Triglycerides, oral testosterone and, 200

TV in bed, sleep and, 344

U

Urinary problems, in menopause, 83

Urinary tract infections, 265

U.S. Pharmacopeia, 336

Uterine cancer

birth control pills and, 330–31

estrogen and, 42, 60, 135, 261, 281

progestin with estrogen

cyclic doses, 299

to lower risk, 42, 72, 136, 261–62,

World Health Organization hip fracture
   study, 168

Y
Yam, wild
  bone health and, 352
  hot flashes and, 338
  vaginal dryness and, 348

ABOUT THE AUTHOR

Tara Parker-Pope has been a professional reporter for 20 years, currently serving as the weekly consumer health columnist for the *Wall Street Journal.* Her special report on the findings of the Women's Health Initiative earned her the Media Award from the North American Menopause Society, as well as the Second Century Award for Excellence in Health Care from the Columbia University School of Nursing. Parker-Pope's professional resume includes tenures with the *Houston Chronicle* and the *Austin American-Statesman.* She also is the author of *Cigarettes: Anatomy of an Industry from Seed to Smoke.* A 1988 graduate of the University of Texas, she currently resides insoutheastern Pennsylvania.

The employees of Thorndike Press hope you have enjoyed this Large Print book. All our Thorndike and Wheeler Large Print titles are designed for easy reading, and all our books are made to last. Other Thorndike Press Large Print books are available at your library, through selected bookstores, or directly from us.

For information about titles, please call:
(800) 223-1244

or visit our Web site at:
http://gale.cengage.com/thorndike

To share your comments, please write:
Publisher
Thorndike Press
295 Kennedy Memorial Drive
Waterville, ME 04901